More praise for *Super Nutrition for Babies*

"The terrible public health experiment of the low-fat, plant-based diet has left our culture in a wreckage of confusion, guilt, and disease. But finally, here is a book for the people who need it most: parents. You only get one chance to grow a child's body, mind, and spirit, and with our traditional food cultures in shreds, parents have been cut adrift in a sea of conflicting advice. Using clear commonsense and basic nutritional concepts, Katherine Erlich and Kelly Genzlinger have written a book that can be an anchor, and then a safe harbor, for parents and babies everywhere."

—Lierre Keith, author of *The Vegetarian Myth: Food, Justice, and Sustainability*

"A clear, practical, and nontrendy guide for parents on how to best feed babies and toddlers, backed by the trifecta of common sense, ancestral wisdom, and sound science. The recommendations accord with Weston A. Price Foundation principles, and are exactly what's needed to get our children off to a good start and to empower their health for life."

—Kaayla T. Daniel, Ph.D., C.C.N., Vice President, Weston A. Price Foundation, and author of *The Whole Soy Story: The Dark Side of America's Favorite Health Food*

"*Super Nutrition for Babies* by Katherine Erlich and Kelly Genzlinger is something that every expectant and new mother and father should read! It gives the correct information for parents on how to bring up healthy, intelligent and robust children. In a world where parents are constantly bombarded by wrong and harmful information, this book is a rare treasure! I congratulate the authors, who write with authority based on solid clinical and practical experience and their work as a medical doctor and a nutritionist—all supported by thorough research and references. I warmly recommend it."

—Natasha Campbell-McBride, M.D., author of *Gut and Psychology Syndrome*

"Erlich and Genzlinger have compiled a wealth of knowledge and experience into a book that is so basic on one hand and so complete and thorough on the other that readers will understand—without difficulty—the concepts and be able to apply them easily. This book is a grand reference book that can be used for many years of a child's life."

—Nancy Appleton, Ph.D., author of *Lick the Sugar Habit*

SUPER NUTRITION

**THE RIGHT WAY
TO FEED YOUR BABY
FOR OPTIMAL HEALTH**

NUTRITION

for babies

Katherine Erlich, M.D. and
Kelly Genzlinger, C.N.C., C.M.T.A.

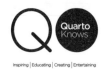

Brimming with creative inspiration, how-to projects, and useful information to enrich your everyday life, Quarto Knows is a favorite destination for those pursuing their interests and passions. Visit our site and dig deeper with our books into your area of interest: Quarto Creates, Quarto Cooks, Quarto Homes, Quarto Lives, Quarto Drives, Quarto Explores, Quarto Gifts, or Quarto Kids.

First published in 2012 by Fair Winds Press,
an imprint of The Quarto Group,
100 Cummings Center, Suite 265-D,
Beverly, MA 01915, USA.
T (978) 282-9590 F (978) 283-2742
www.QuartoKnows.com

Fair Winds Press titles are also available at discount for retail, wholesale, promotional, and bulk purchase. For details, contact the Special Sales Manager by email at specialsales@quarto.com or by mail at The Quarto Group, Attn: Special Sales Manager, 401 Second Avenue North, Suite 310, Minneapolis, MN 55401, USA.

19 18   17 18 19 20

ISBN: 978-1-59233-503-9

Digital edition published in 2012
eISBN: 978-159-233-503-9

Library of Congress Cataloging-in-Publication Data
Genzlinger, Kelly.
    Super nutrition for babies : the right way to feed your baby for optimal health / Kelly Genzlinger, Kathy Erlich
        p. cm.
    Includes bibliographical references and index.
    ISBN 978-1-59233-503-9 (pbk.) -- ISBN 1-59233-503-9 (pbk.)
    1. Infants--Nutrition. I. Erlich, Kathy. II. Title.
    RJ216.G3745 2012
    641.5'6222--dc23

                                    2011041666

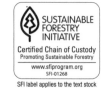

SUSTAINABLE
FORESTRY
INITIATIVE

Certified Chain of Custody
Promoting Sustainable Forestry
www.sfiprogram.org
SFI-01268

SFI label applies to the text stock

Cover and Book design by Kathie Alexander

Printed and bound in USA

Foreword

Super Nutrition for Babies is a much-needed book. Parents are confused about food and often do not have the appropriate knowledge to make the best food choices for their children. Now they have a book that guides them toward making good food decisions.

Conventional medicine makes little mention of the importance of educating parents about how to properly feed their children. Simple dietary changes that emphasize eating nutrient-rich foods would do more than any medicine or vaccine to improve a child's ability to reach their potential. In fact, educating parents about the optimal way to feed their children should be the first item discussed in the prenatal visit. *Super Nutrition for Babies* provides the optimal dietary advice that gives children the best chance to reach their true potential.

Health care for children is a disaster. What is health care for children? Conventional medicine spends untold amounts of moneys vaccinating children for numerous illnesses. And yes, many childhood illnesses have declined due to vaccinations. However, epidemic numbers of children are suffering from a host of chronic illnesses such as autism, cancer, obesity, and ADHD.

In the United States, for instance, far more money is spent on health care than any other Western country. Currently, more than 16 percent of the U.S.'s gross domestic product is spent on health care. Unfortunately, spending large sums of money on health care has not provided better health indices. As compared to other Western countries, the U.S. ranks at the bottom of nearly every health indicator. There is more chronic illness, more heart attacks, and generally poorer health when compared to other Western countries. However, it is not just U.S. children that are suffering. All Western countries are seeing dramatic increases of chronic childhood diseases such as autism, ADD/ADHD, and cancer.

Is there an underlying theme behind the declining health of our children? It is not as simple as spending more money. Every country in the world is under strain due to budgetary constraints. In the case of children's health needs, one inexpensive way to improve the health of children is to feed them nutritious food. This would go a long way to helping the world overcome its health-care crises. This process can be started by following the healthy dietary principles outlined in *Super Nutrition for Babies*.

I have been practicing holistic medicine for nearly twenty years. I have seen the consequences of feeding children a poor diet full of refined and devitalized foods. Feeding children a devitalized diet leads to devitalized children that will not reach their potential and suffer from myriad health issues.

My experience has clearly shown that the pathway to optimal health for us all is to eat a healthy diet. The pathway to raising a child who can achieve her full potential is to provide the child with a diet that supplies all of the valuable nutrients needed to help optimize their brain function. A healthy diet can also help the child optimize her immune and hormonal systems as well as all the other organs of the body.

Katherine Erlich, M.D., and Kelly Genzlinger, C.N.C., C.M.T.A, have written a must-read book for everyone who has children and for those who are thinking of starting a family. There is no doubt that the younger your child is when you begin optimizing his/her diet, the greater the tools he or she will have to succeed. These tools include vitamins, minerals, enzymes, and fatty acids. The Western diet is lacking in each of these vital items. For nearly twenty years, I have been testing children (and adults) for various nutritional levels. Eating a devitalized diet, full of refined foods, leads to multiple nutritional deficiencies and poor brain function.

We can and should do more for our children. It starts with mothers eating healthier diets. Erlich and Genzlinger discuss this in chapter 7. They point out that eating refined sugar and soy is not a good idea for mothers.

I see the benefits of properly feeding children. These children have less allergies, behavioral problems, chronic illness, depression, fatigue, and digestive problems. Furthermore, children fed a whole foods program as outlined in *Super Nutrition for Babies* have stronger immune systems.

It makes sense. If you supply the body with the correct nutrients it can do wonderful things. Just as you fuel your car with appropriate gas in order to optimize its function, we need to fuel our children with appropriate food. Children should eat whole food that is nutritious and supplies the body with the appropriate nutrients to maintain optimal function. In addition, educating children about which foods are healthy and which are not will help future generations. Erlich and Genzlinger have provided us with a blueprint for feeding our children the perfect diet. I highly recommend this book for everyone interested in improving their family's health.

DAVID BROWNSTEIN, M.D., *is a board certified family practitioner and medical director of the Center for Holistic Medicine (West Bloomfield, Michigan). He is the author of ten books, including* **Iodine: Why You Need It, Why You Can't Live Without It** *and* **Overcoming Thyroid Disorders.** *To learn more, visit www.drbrownstein.com.*

Dedication

To Babies:

This book is dedicated to all the babies being born everywhere. To you, we say: "You deserve a fair chance to be fully healthy. You are designed to be that way, down to your very cells. You are perfect." Yet despite your potential for perfection, you are among a generation of babies being shortchanged of this healthy birthright.

To Parents:

We acknowledge that, while joyous, having a baby these days is also scary. Health threats are increasing on many fronts; one of the goals of this book is to give you critical knowledge and resources so you can help your children live long, healthy, and happy lives—ideally, preventing modern illnesses. We're writing this book to support you as you support your child.

We hope you are encouraged that your child can be protected from many common modern diseases. There are ways to safeguard him and improve his odds in favor of health—traditional ways to nourish your child that will likely resonate with you and ring true on a deep level. By providing the purest, most nutritious, and least-toxic foods, you have the power to give your baby a solid foundation in health. With the guidance provided in this book, you will learn how to help him be the most resilient, strongest, happiest, and healthiest child possible.

To Pediatricians:

For those of you who have ever felt frustrated or helpless in caring for even one child suffering with chronic or recurrent illness, we also dedicate this book to you. We hope that this book will be an additional resource in assisting you in the treatment of your patients, and family members, about whom you care so dearly.

Contents

Introduction
Children's New Health Concerns

We are so excited for you—new parents! There isn't a more magical time than welcoming your little one into your life and cultivating a family dynamic around your newest member. Time passes quickly in the first two years, each day bringing fresh wonders as his abilities to smile, coo, clutch, crawl, walk, and speak all continue to develop.

We wish you congratulations during this life-changing and memorable chapter in your life. During this time of early parenthood, you too will develop new abilities—those of mother or father, protector, provider, and caregiver. Feed-ing is but one aspect of how you will care for your baby, and this book will provide you with the best guidance available in terms of when, how, why, and what to feed him.

New Concerns: The 3Cs

All parents wish for their children to have optimal health. But today we have more to fear in terms of pediatric health than parents did just two or three generations ago. In fact, back when your great-grandparents were giving birth to your grandparents, the general public had never heard of autism, celiac disease was incredibly rare, and peanuts were synonymous with baseball games and springtime. Cancer, type 2 diabetes, heart disease, arthritis, and obesity were diseases of the *aged*. Just a few generations ago, children, by and large, were healthy, strong, and robust.

We see children's health getting worse with each subsequent generation. Our children today are at grave risk, and parents' worries are both many and valid. Tragically, the most recent generation of babies is slated to have *shorter* life spans than their parents. *This is unacceptable!*

Many of the conditions kids face today are new and thus, are issues for which parents can no longer call upon the wisdom of mothers or grandmothers (who have no experience with "stimming" or EpiPens or nebulizers). Parents, perhaps even you, are turning to other parents in support groups and are becoming researchers, analysts, and metabolic "specialists" themselves in their quest to find help for their children.

As such, we recognize the following illnesses as being *Contemporary Chronic Childhood* conditions—the "3Cs":

▶ Autistic spectrum disorders
▶ Allergies, eczema
▶ Asthma
▶ Attention deficit disorders and learning disabilities
▶ Recurrent pain disorders (headaches. abdominal pain, joint pain)
▶ Emotional, mood, and behavioral disorders (anxiety disorders, depression, bipolar disorder)
▶ Digestive disorders (irritable and inflammatory bowel disorders, gastroesophageal reflux, eosinophilic esophagitis, and gastroenteritis)
▶ Autoimmune conditions (celiac disease, type 1 diabetes, thyroid disorders)
▶ Obesity, metabolic syndrome, and type 2 diabetes
▶ Tooth decay
▶ Cancer

Many of the 3C conditions are directly *caused* by our modern world, which is full of toxins and nutrient-poor foods (that are themselves a source of toxins). These toxins and deficiencies cripple many areas of the body, causing multiple symptoms and resulting in a veritable puzzle for modern medicine. Often, highly specialized conventional medical models fail to see the whole, for their strict focus on each of the parts. Looking at the *whole* child through a *holistic* perspective is often necessary to piece all the symptoms together when it comes to the 3Cs.

Though conventional medicine claims most of the 3C conditions are incurable, this isn't the last word. The good news is that most children with 3C conditions can improve. But more important, by following a program of Super Nutrition—the program you're holding in your hands— these problems can be *prevented and often cured*.

It boils down to this: Poor health comes from poor foods. Undernourished children are more vulnerable to infection, more susceptible to toxins and cancer, and more likely to develop learning, attention, and behavioral problems.

Since you're reading this book, we know that you want more for your child than what today's statistics promise. Instead of worrying about the bad and just hoping for good, you are taking control of your child's health destiny. Food is one of the most powerful tools you have to protect, preserve, and ensure your baby's health and well-being. In the coming chapters, we'll introduce the concept of Super Nutrition and explain how providing foods that are rich in critical nutrients, as well as reducing toxins, will enable your baby's body to function optimally. We'll focus on what you can proactively *do* to create a fundamental base of good health for your baby and significantly increase the odds of your baby living a long, happy, and *healthy* life.

A Better Way

When researchers and anthropologists study nonindustrialized cultures, they find that they are often free of heart disease, cancer, infertility, emotional and behavioral disturbances, birth defects, diabetes, autism, life-threatening allergies, and other afflictions that are commonly accepted in our culture today. Even in just the last generation, we have seen a marked statistical increase in these conditions that experts remark are not attributable to better testing, awareness, or diagnosis. In fact, the 3Cs were so rare in preindustrialized cultures that these relatively new conditions are often called *Diseases of Civilization*.

This is significant. Research corroborates that when we modernize and "industrialize" our foods (and our environment), we increasingly get Diseases of Civilization with each generation. This is very important when you consider what to feed your baby because food is the most significant "environmental" component in his life. Diet can make a positive impact on your baby's health and development—or be a major detriment to his health.

Though many attest that life was much shorter "back then," it is actually true that many primitive cultures, such as the Russian Georgians, Pakistani Hunza, and Ecuadorian Vilcabamba peoples, heralded healthy octo-, nono-, and even centenarians. It was once believed that cancer and diabetes developed only because "modern man" was living longer. We've since learned, however, that these are not just "adult-onset" diseases, but rather are diseases of industrialization—as now even our children increasingly suffer with them.

Many preindustrialized cultures held certain indigenous foods sacred; science proves these to be particularly nutritious foods. We'll show you which foods these are, and how to prepare them, in the chapters to come. Many of our grandparents and great-grandparents also recognized the power of food, feeding their families organ meats and spooning out cod liver oil. Somehow this knowledge has slowly faded away, while processed foods have taken center stage.

Even as recently as when our parents were children, they had far fewer toxic exposures. They did not have genetically modified foods or high fructose corn syrup; they had fewer pesticides and far fewer antibiotics given to their food animals (and themselves); they were given significantly fewer vaccines, had no bromine in their bread, less radiation in their skies, fewer chemicals on their skin, no cell phones or laptops, and far more sun exposure and daily exercise. Their diets were fresher, more local, more pure, less processed, and substantially more nutritious.

Traditional wisdom, passed down through countless generations, directed parents to feed their babies the most nutrient-rich foods available, which included the meat, fat, and organs from poultry (including ducks and geese), red meat (including lamb and wild game), and fish and shellfish. Eggs, milk, raw dairy, bone broths, and even insects were also commonly found in preindustrialized diets. These foods were accompanied by select, *seasonal* fruits, veggies, nuts, seeds, and occasionally specially prepared grains and beans.

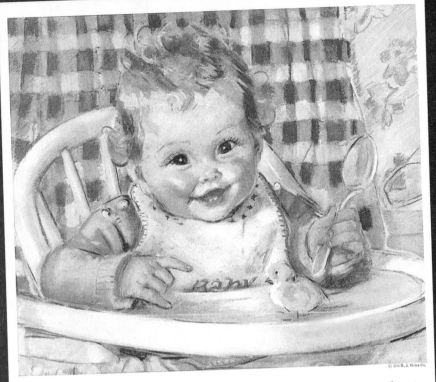

Only the Best is Good Enough for Baby!

BABY is the most important member of any household. His health should be—*must be*—protected at any cost! "Bargains" in food should not be for him—when absolute safety is so easy to buy and costs so little!

In most stores Heinz Strained Foods cost no more than ordinary brands. Each tin bears both the Seal of Acceptance of the American Medical Association Committee on Foods and the world-renowned Heinz 57 Seal! No other strained foods are more distinguished!

You use Heinz products at your table because the name Heinz assures dependable food quality—purity and appetizing taste. Isn't your baby entitled to the same consideration? Especially when it's so easy to let him have Heinz foods too!

Even among the smallest youngsters many detect the taste difference in Heinz Strained Foods . . . *prefer* Heinz! They enjoy the taste

of "garden freshness", the rich, natural color, the wholesome goodness that's cooked *in*—never cooked out. And Heinz Strained Foods are just the right consistency—neither too fine to be palatable nor too coarse for easy digesting. Heinz cooking methods, too, conserve a higher vitamin content than is usually possible with ordinary home-kitchen methods.

Insist on Heinz Strained Foods! Give baby the same *quality* in foods that you enjoy. Give him Heinz—the strained foods that he *enjoys* eating! Let your physician name the varieties best suited for your baby.

Send For This Baby Diet Book
This new book "*Modern Guardians of Your Baby's Health*", contains many up-to-date facts regarding the various vitamins and mineral salts. Also information on infant care and feeding. Send labels from 3 tins of Heinz Strained Foods or 10 cents. Address H. J. Heinz Co., Dep., D307, Pittsburgh, Pa.

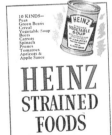

10 KINDS—
Peas
Green Beans
Cereal
Vegetable Soup
Beets
Carrots
Spinach
Prunes
Tomatoes
Apricots &
Apple Sauce

HEINZ STRAINED FOODS

We've placed advertisements, such as this one from 1936, throughout the book illustrating what babies were fed in the 1930s, '40s, and '50s, as well as what appealed to parents who selected and judged foods based on what their mothers had fed them. (The mid-last century heralded the introduction of the first commercial baby foods—before then, babies were only fed homemade foods). We haven't included these ads as a way to recommend canned and jarred baby foods, but instead we intend to demonstrate that, indeed, our recommendations are throwbacks to earlier generations' methods of feeding babies and toddlers. These were decades in which deathly allergies, asthma, autism, attention problems, depression, diabetes, and even obesity were extremely rare in children. We intend for these ads to be reminders of the nutritional guidance of our great-grandparents and ancestors and a way of feeding that we now know was more protective than today's dietary regimen. As this ad suggests, your baby's "health should be—*must be*—protected at any cost!" It states: "'Bargains' in food should not be for him . . . " and we attest: nor should compromised nutrition—in the name of convenience. This ad appealed to the wisdom of generations ago, that babies should be fed foods of sufficient "purity" and with "garden freshness," "natural color," and "wholesome goodness," which comes from "higher vitamin content."

It is time to feed our babies differently than our current standard. Instead of relying on our newfangled "Franken-foods" of industrialization, we recommend going back to the more natural foods of preindustrialized peoples that did a far better job of keeping the children of our ancestors healthy.

Cutting Edge, but Traditionally Sound

Can food really protect your child? Hippocrates said, "Let food be thy medicine, and let thy medicine be food." Unfortunately, this ancient wisdom has been lost in the name of food companies' media storms, advertising blitzes, and continual tsunami of consumer data. Let's admit it: We've been relying on marketers to tell us what is healthy, to teach us how to feed our kids, and even to provide doctors with their "nutritional education" (which is lacking in conventional medical schools). But the truth is, those marketers and their advertisements aren't motivated to make healthy kids—they're driven to sell products and make profit.

To ensure the proper health of our children, we must resist being seduced by convenience-based processed foods. Too often parents focus on making sure their children get *enough calories*, rather than focusing on the *nutrients* their kids most need. And too often we say we're too busy for anything but fast food, or packaged food, or "junk" food. Yet, it is *whole* food that heals, *real* food that protects, and *traditional* food that nourishes.

We realize that what we present here is unconventional and . . . well, *different*. Yet a decade of working with patients and finding considerable rates of success in improving health and quality of life for babies and young children—and ameliorating root-cause issues relating to the 3Cs—has incited us to spread the word. What we offer—*the fundamentals of Super Nutrition feeding for babies*—works differently than "normal" baby feeding. It serves to safeguard health and normal development, as well as to restore quality of life in children with modern, chronic cognitive, emotional, and physical illnesses.

In addition to our own practical, personal, and professional application of Super Nutrition, we have extensively researched and studied the findings of world-renowned experts, who have also found remarkable success through such feeding principles. Though our approach to feeding babies is far from mainstream, it is both cutting-edge and traditionally sound. Super Nutrition is a way of feeding your child that gives the best nutrition for optimal development, cognitively and physically, *and* is protective against illnesses and 3C conditions. Do this for your child and you'll be optimizing his/her health *now* and years from now.

Implementing and practicing Super Nutrition is not easy—and we're saying this right from the get-go, just so there's no confusion. If you want easy, stick with the Standard American Diet—its entire premise is convenience. If, however, you want optimal health for your baby, then you'll have to give up some conveniences. Our program is comprised of special foods and purposeful ways of preparing and making meals; therefore, special attention and time is required. We provide some tricks and guidance to make things easier, though, and the more you do it, the easier it will become.

And there's a bonus: Most of the parents we've worked with who start spending more time practicing Super Nutrition find a deep sense of satisfaction and fulfillment that they don't find anywhere else—it is one of knowing that they are truly nourishing their children, a gift no one else can give.

While you might be excited to "get going" with Super Nutrition and want to flip to the age-appropriate chapter for your child, we hope you'll read this book in full. In the first chapter, we lay the groundwork for our feeding program—the *what*, the *how*, and even more important, the *why*. We'll show you why our way is a better way of feeding your baby—as well as explain how current mainstream feeding trends aren't all they're cracked up to be. We'll share with you our Super Nutrition food categories and show you how easy it is to make nutritionally sound selections for your child if you keep these categories in mind. We'll also discuss our four pillars of Super Nutrition—improving digestion, eliminating toxins, safeguarding immunity, and eating nutrient-worthy, whole foods—and what they can mean for your baby's health. In chapters 2 through 6, we'll break them out and examine each pillar in more detail.

The chapters have been organized to follow the growth, age, and stages of development of your child, beginning with his first introduction to food and coinciding with our program's foundational pillars. Though the recipes that accompany each chapter are specific for the age of your child at that time, the nutritional benefits cannot be outgrown. Thus, you can use the recipes and information gained in each chapter for your entire family.

If you're reading this book before your bundle of joy has even arrived, we salute you! You cannot begin protective nutrition early enough. Super Nutrition for your baby begins with you—beginning with what you "feed" your baby in utero to what you eat while producing milk to feed your baby. (Our nursing dietary guidelines in chapter 7 are also ideal for eating during pregnancy.) But as we also recognize that some parents will not or cannot nurse, we've included a special chapter, chapter 8, on making your own formula that closely mimics the nutrition found in mom's milk and is so much more protective and nourishing than what you'd find in a canister.

Throughout each of the chapters we've added tips, tricks, and ideas to help ease you into implementing our program—look for the boxes called "Mom to Mom." Finally, we've included a thorough resources section that includes essential where-to-buy information on many of the ingredients we recommend as well as countless books and websites to turn to for further information.

Super Nutrition for Babies will help you reap the benefits that traditional foods can provide. It will show you how to make better food choices for your baby and how to prepare those foods so that they can be most nourishing. Your baby deserves nothing but the *best*!

1

Baby Feeding Fundamentals

Nutrition Is Necessary for Health

Most of the great healthy-baby feeding books have a lot in common. They tell you to choose organic produce, alert you to choking hazards, urge you to make your own baby food, encourage breast-feeding, and provide you with some developmental expectations for your child related to feeding. We'll tell you all of this too, but we're also going to provide you with much, much more.

Our recommendations are quite different from mainstream advice—this is because feeding children as we currently do is not good enough. We'll tell you why and offer you much better options—what we call the Super Nutrition Baby Feeding Program.

These feeding guidelines will not just provide your baby with the ability to survive but will ensure she *thrives*. We recommend feeding your baby in a way that coincides with how her body works, considering her unique nutrient needs *as a growing baby*. (As you'll learn, most modern feeding suggestions surprisingly do *not* consider these facts!)

Our Super Nutrition program builds superhealthy babies. And today a healthy baby is not a certainty, as evidenced by the increasing numbers of children with chronic health issues. Diet and nutrition *can* make a tremendous difference to your baby's current and future health.

A Tidal Wave of Disease

Despite the efforts of well-intentioned parents everywhere, following the advice of doctors and the media, "healthy" feeding over the last twenty to thirty years hasn't helped to slow the development of chronic childhood illness. Rather, chronic childhood illness has been on a steep *rise*. We call this scourge of *Contemporary Chronic Childhood* maladies "3C" conditions, and they include autism spectrum disorders; allergies, eczema, and asthma; attention deficit disorders and learning disabilities; emotional, mood, and behavioral disorders; recurrent pain disorders; metabolic syndrome, obesity, and autoimmune diseases; digestive disorders; tooth decay; and cancer.

We consider the 3C conditions *contemporary* because they are relatively modern illnesses that were exceedingly rare in past generations and in fact, nonexistent in preindustrialized populations. They are *chronic* because they aren't an acute problem, like pneumonia, but are instead those that chip away at health every day and are often considered incurable. They are designated as *childhood* conditions because they primarily (and sometimes uniquely) affect children, are increasing in prevalence in childhood, and some (like type 2 diabetes, metabolic syndrome, depression, and heart disease) are new to childhood, as previously they only affected adults.

Not only are the 3C conditions on the rise in children, but many, such as obesity, autism, asthma, and diabetes, are increasing at such rates as to be called epidemics. While hundreds of baby-feeding books, pediatricians, and government agencies are telling parents how to feed their babies, none of the current advice has done *anything* to stop this tidal wave of disease in children.

Children born today face the following unfortunate statistical realities:

▸ One in five children have allergies.
▸ One in twelve have food allergies.
▸ One in ten have asthma.
▸ One in three have either ADHD, allergies, asthma, or autism.
▸ Almost one in ten show signs of depression.
▸ More than one in one hundred are diagnosed with autism.
▸ One in thirty-eight have autistic traits.

Assuming the diet and environment of children remains constant, for those born this century:

▸ Nearly one in two will become obese or overweight.
▸ One in three will eventually suffer with diabetes.

What's worse is that these disease rates have been progressively increasing over the years. "If these trends continue," fears William Sears, M.D., pediatrician and author of more than forty books on children's health, "America's children face a future filled with sickness rather than health, of weakness rather than strength, of sadness rather than happiness."

Introducing Super Nutrition

With this book as your guide, we will empower you to put the odds in your favor for preventing your baby from developing such 3C conditions, despite the statistics. Our way to do that is with *Super Nutrition*. Super Nutrition is the term we've coined to describe a purposeful way of selecting, preparing, and combining foods; using specific supplements; and purposefully avoiding other foodstuffs in such a way as to be protective of health. Ideally, these choices will result in the *prevention* of chronic and degenerative disease in your child.

Put another way, Super Nutrition is a mindful way of nourishing children to safeguard them from modern-day illness and to preserve their chance for genuine health. Our feeding program, therefore, is *preventive*. This means that by feeding your baby following our Super Nutrition method, you can *protect* her from the very real, very scary, and very tragic 3C conditions.

You might wonder how the same feeding program can protect against such a wide array of illness. There are significant commonalities in the underlying causes of many of the 3C conditions. So even though they don't seem to have a lot in common—allergies seem different from autism, and asthma seems different from learning disabilities, which seem far removed from diabetes or autoimmune conditions—the 3C conditions actually have two very important things in common: They are caused or made worse by nutrient deficiencies, and they are caused or made worse by toxic overload.

Both of these contributing components are *environmental* factors of diet and lifestyle. Unfortunately, most people don't give much credit to the role environment plays in health. Perhaps you too think that genetics or luck will determine the state of your baby's health. Previously, even experts hypothesized that health was equally determined by nurture (environment) and nature (genetics). But due to the findings of the Human Genome Project and the scientific field of epigenetics, we now know *there is a*

difference between our DNA (with which we are born) *and what actually comes to be* (how the genes are expressed) —and that difference is our *environment*.

Professor Jose M. Ordovas, Ph.D., director of the Nutrition and Genomics program at Tufts University and a recognized expert in the field of nutrigenomics, attests that *no more* than 25 percent of health is actually because of hard-coded genetics. This means *at least* 75 percent of health is up to environmental factors (and many experts think their influence is even greater!). Environment— because it influences genes—plays a far greater role in our health than does just "genetics."

This is great news! It means that *you* hold most of your baby's health in your hands because you have significant control over her environment. Even if she has "bad" genetics (or genetic susceptibility) that sets her up for autism, diabetes, obesity, learning disabilities, or emotional disorders, *it is most often* not *her genes, but rather her environment that will determine whether she actually ever gets any of these conditions.*

IMPACT OF DIET AND LIFESTYLE ON HEALTH

For babies, *diet* is, by and large, the most impactful environmental factor when it comes to influencing health. The foods selected, their source, their preparation, their timing of introduction, their quality, and their combination are all important in the protection of health ("good" gene expression) or the development of disease ("bad" gene expression). *Simply put: Good food keeps good genes* on *and keeps bad-disease genes turned* off.

In fact, as you will see, "typical" feeding practices and kid-friendly foods not only aren't protecting our children, but rather are actually *contributing* to the development and prevalence of chronic disease. Truth be told, we see modern food and conveniences as an attack, or veritable war, against children's health.

Enemies and Allies in the War on Children's Health

The fundamental premise for our Super Nutrition Baby Feeding Program is putting protective nutrition into practical application so that parents and children can reap the benefits. In this war on children's health, we have identified "Allies" and "Enemies." While the Standard American Diet (SAD) is sadly light in the former and heavy in the latter, our program inherently incorporates plenty of Allies and keeps Enemies at bay.

SUPER NUTRITION'S ALLIED ARMED FORCES

Your Allies are the diet and lifestyle choices you make that will work to protect your baby from the 3Cs—they are essential to Super Nutrition. Allies include not just what you choose to put into your baby's mouth but also what you include in her life to bolster her internal defenses, like good bacteria, sunshine, clean water, and fresh air.

Anti-inflammation. One of the fundamental problems seen in children with the 3Cs is underlying inflammation of various tissues and organs, most notably the brain. Calming this inflammation is a key factor in preventing disease. To tame the flames of inflammation, it is important to support

intestinal health, minimize toxic overload, optimize nutrient balances, and bolster immune function—all of which are key to Super Nutrition.

Proper digestion and digestive aids. Children with the 3Cs often have digestive problems. Therefore, it is critical to aim for complete protein digestion as well as adequate stomach acid to ensure proper nutrition is obtained from foods; it's also essential to prevent a variety of tummy troubles, from constipation to diarrhea. Additionally, improving digestion will avoid the consequences of undigested foods, such as food allergies, bad bacterial overgrowth, and mood alterations. (More on digestion in chapter 2.)

Healthy gut ecosystem and intestinal wall. When the tissue of the intestinal wall is well nourished and coated with beneficial bacteria, it creates a powerful barrier to the "outside" world. When gut tissue is malnourished, it is weak and thin—a veritable haven for pathogenic bacteria and yeasts. Proper nourishment will ensure that your baby's intestinal tissue is healthy and capable of protecting her from undigested proteins and pathogens that could otherwise gain access to her bloodstream and brain.

Clean water. As the average human body is more than 60 percent water, closer to 75 percent for infants, your baby's growing body is, in part, built based on the caliber of water you provide for her. Using filtered water, when your baby is ready, will help to ensure that the water she drinks functions appropriately as a cleanser rather than a source of toxins.

Vitamins and minerals. Vitamins and minerals are called micronutrients because we need them in smaller amounts than the macronutrients fat, carbohydrate, and protein. But just because they are needed in small amounts doesn't make them less important. Tiny, trace quantities of certain minerals enable the body to run its complex biochemical processes. Similarly, vitamins and minerals are also called *coenzymes* and act as critical helpers in making certain processes in the body function effectively and efficiently. Every biochemical process in the body requires vitamins, minerals, and enzymes. In addition to ensuring the body "works" properly, nutrients are the building blocks for your baby's tissues, bones, and organs. Small nutrient deficiencies can cause *big* problems. Whole foods are your best source of nutrients.

Detoxification. Nature designed the body with an amazing capability to cope with damaging substances. However, while the human body evolved dealing with limited *natural* toxins, today we have *more* and *different* toxins than ever before. Furthermore, babies' young bodies and systems are far more vulnerable to toxins than are adults'. While toxins are more likely to overwhelm a body that lacks nutrients, a well-nourished body fortunately can cope far better. By providing nutritious foods, you will support your baby's ability to detoxify and thus minimize the effects of these toxins. (More in chapter 3.)

Healing ("Super POWER") foods. Certain foods provide optimal nutrition to support immunity, detoxification, formation of organs, and the function of many systems in the body. These foods have been shown to protect and preserve pristine health. When abandoned in the diet, their absence has been associated with an increase in chronic disease, deformity, and degeneration. When replaced, these foods have the power to actually restore health. Thus, we have categorized these protective, nutrient-rich, healing foods as Super POWER foods. As most of them are no longer common in today's diet, we've provided recipes throughout the book, starting in chapter 2, to help both you and your baby work these POWERful foods into your diets.

Real foods. Real foods—as we define them—are those that are as Nature designed them. That means they exist in their whole form: full-fat milk, not skimmed; unrefined salt, not just sodium chloride; whole grains, not stripped apart and bleached. Real foods do not have elements that are refined, as in sugar, where "sweetness" is extracted from whole cane, beet, or corn. Real foods do not have unnatural ingredients, like additives, preservatives, colorings, flavorings, or texturizers. Real foods come from animals who naturally graze on pastures, enjoying fresh air and sunlight, and who are never given pharmaceutical drugs or synthetic hormones. Real foods are grown in organic soil free of pesticides, chemicals, and nitrates, where nutrients are replenished through natural sources such as manure and crop rotation rather than chemical fertilizer. While real foods are much more than just "organic," organic is a great place to start. Real foods are pure, are worthy of your baby's body, and ideally support health. (We cover real, pure foods in greater depth in chapter 3.)

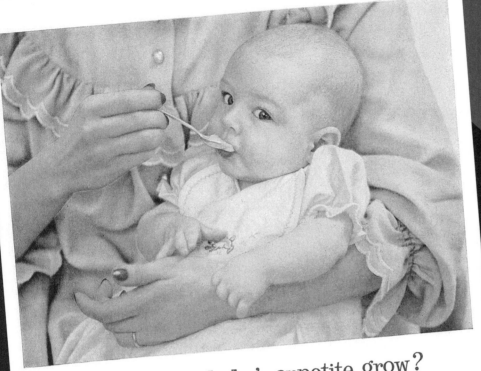

What makes baby's appetite grow?

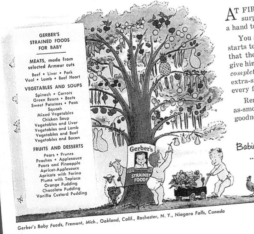

GERBER'S STRAINED FOODS FOR BABY

MEATS, made from selected Armour cuts
Beef • Liver • Pork
Veal • Lamb • Beef Heart

VEGETABLES AND SOUPS
Spinach • Carrots
Green Beans • Beets
Sweet Potatoes • Peas
Squash
Mixed Vegetables
Chicken Soup
Vegetables and Liver
Vegetables and Lamb
Vegetables and Beef
Vegetables and Bacon

FRUITS AND DESSERTS
Pears • Prunes
Peaches • Applesauce
Pears and Pineapple
Apricot-Applesauce
Apricots with Farina
Plums with Tapioca
Orange Pudding
Chocolate Pudding
Vanilla Custard Pudding

AT FIRST, your cherub's hunger just naturally grows! But it's surprising how a healthy appetite can lag—unless Mommy takes a hand to keep baby really *interested* in eating.

You see, by the time your baby starts on strained foods, he also starts to develop a greater sense of color and taste. So you'll notice that the more different varieties of Gerber's Strained Foods you give him, the more his appetite perks up. For Gerber's make a really *complete* choice for your little one's meal-times. And Gerber's take extra-special care to keep the tempting, natural color of each and every food . . . and the appetizing, individual true flavor, too!

Remember that Gerber's are also famous for the smooth-as-smooth texture that your baby enjoys . . . the wholesome goodness that you and your doctor look for.

Babies are our business . . . our only business!

 Gerber's BABY FOODS

4 CEREALS • 40 STRAINED & JUNIOR FOODS • 10 MEATS

Gerber's Baby Foods, Fremont, Mich., Oakland, Calif., Rochester, N. Y., Niagara Falls, Canada

Supplements. Supplements are ideally just that: "supplemental" to a nourishing diet. Food provides nutrients in their most absorbable form, acting synergistically to provide the best support for the body. However, many factors in our modern lifestyle make our nutrient needs greater than ever before. But despite our elevated need for nutrients, foods today have far *fewer* nutrients than they once did due to processing, refining, and depleted soils. Thus, supplements are often beneficial to fill a nutrient void or to support a metabolic blockage, but they can never replace good nutrition.

Antioxidants. Antioxidants are nutrients that protect your cells against free radicals, which cause damage to the body that results in inflammation and other problems. Antioxidant nutrients work to temper the larger load of free-radical onslaught common today and reduce the damage they can cause.

Probiotics. *Probiotics* is another term for beneficial bacteria, which serve untold health functions in the body. Whenever beneficial bacteria are destroyed (such as from antibiotics or steroids) or significantly limited, the entire gut ecosystem can be affected and the integrity of the intestinal lining damaged. Maintaining healthy gut flora will protect against a damaged or "leaky" gut, thus minimizing the risk of allergies, of mood alterations, and illness from infection. (More on probiotics in chapter 4.)

Strong immune system. The immune system has several levels of protection that it invokes to maintain health, as well as prevent illness. The first line of defense is the digestive system! Deeper support comes from the cellular immune "army," who are kept strong with adequate nutrients. Our baby-feeding regimen provides the best possible support for your baby's immune system troops. (We'll tell you more about immunity boosting in chapter 4.)

Sunshine, fresh air, and physical activity. Once the hallmark of childhood, running around the block, drawing hopscotch with chalk, climbing trees, exploring, building forts, jumping rope, and riding bikes have given way to TV, video games, computers, cell phones, and even baby-oriented "learning" DVDs. It is a different world for the youth of today than even when we were children. By encouraging sun exposure, movement, and fresh air, you will improve immune function, detoxification, and your child's overall health as she grows.

THE ENEMIES THAT ATTACK YOUR CHILD'S HEALTH

While just supplying her body with Allies will help your baby be stronger, there are Enemies lurking about that can quickly combine and create cumulative damage, overwhelming the Allies rather effectively. *What makes Enemies particularly powerful is that they are insidious—part of "normal" diet and lifestyle for kids*—and they're increasingly prevalent. While it's impossible to avoid all Enemies, becoming aware of them and reducing exposure to them will minimize their impact on your baby.

Toxins. Toxins include pesticides, pollution, heavy metals, medications, industrial waste, chemicals (found in common items from cleaning and hygiene products to canned and processed foods to tap water), dyes, artificial ingredients, preservatives, and even animal foods (such as

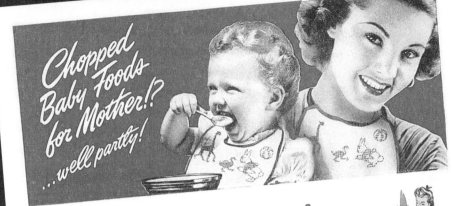

Chopped Baby Foods for Mother!? ...well partly!

1 Of course, you know that Gerber's Chopped (Junior) Foods are for babies who have outgrown Strained Foods and are still not quite ready for family meals. Mothers don't eat them. But mothers buy them and serve them, and they do appreciate little thoughtful conveniences ...

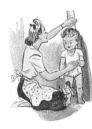

2 ...like, for instance, the shiny little cans Gerber's Chopped Foods come packed in. In the first place, they cost not a whit more than the Strained Foods cans. Which is exclusively a Gerber idea, and we'll bet it's the first thing about baby you paid even less for than you expected!

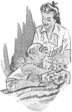

3 What's more, the small size supplies an average portion (along with the other foods in baby's meal) without tiresome left-overs. Saves fuss and refrigerator space, and gives baby a bright new dish to look forward to every day. The scrumptious taste of these home-grown vegetables and meat combinations helps eliminate left-overs too.

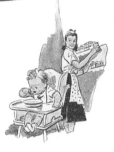

4 Finally, your doctor will want you to make the change to Chopped Foods *gradually*. Having them in the same-size, same-price can makes it simple. Just include a can or two in the batch of Strained Foods—and you don't have to be a genius at mental arithmetic to figure the total price, either! Gerber Products Co., Fremont, Michigan.

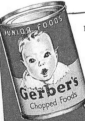

Be sure to ask your doctor about the proper time to start Gerber's Chopped Foods. No need to ask him how baby will take to them, though. My own did, with gusto! And I assure you, they're as pure, wholesome and nourishing as even a mother could wish.

Mrs. Dan Gerber

TEN TEMPTING DISHES FOR YOUR TODDLER:
VEGETABLE AND BEEF · VEGETABLE AND LAMB · VEGETABLE AND LIVER
CREAMED POTATOES · CHOPPED SPINACH · CHOPPED GREEN BEANS · CHOPPED CARROTS
CHICKEN, RICE, CELERY · PINEAPPLE-RICE PUDDING · APPLE-PRUNE-TAPIOCA PUDDING

...by the makers of **Gerber's** *Baby Foods*

CEREALS · STRAINED FOODS · CHOPPED FOODS

◀ As this 1942 ad states: "Gerber's Chopped [Junior] Foods are for babies who . . . are still not quite ready for family meals." They have a "scrumptious taste" of "home-grown vegetables and meat combinations." Dishes included "vegetables and beef," "vegetables and lamb," and "vegetables and liver." Such wise meals are not based on carbs and don't include grains such as noodles, rice, or cereal.

arsenic in poultry from chicken feed and mercury in meat from cattle's grain-based feed). Toxins accumulate in the body and disrupt normal metabolic activity. Many children suffer from a reduced ability to eliminate toxic elements entering the body—due to genetic problems or insufficient nutrients to help enzymes do the job. Toxins then accumulate, crippling various organs and systems in the body and brain. At high-enough doses, many of them are lethal, but even at lower doses, they cause much trouble with normal functioning and development.

With the level of toxic exposure children are unfortunately assaulted with these days, it is more important than ever to conscientiously reduce and remove toxins from your baby's environment and food supply. Understanding what toxins she is likely to encounter will help you to reduce them. The lower the toxic exposure, the less the burden on the body, and thus the easier it is for Super Nutrition to help your baby achieve and maintain optimal heath.

Sugar and refined grains. Present in the daily fare of most children, sugar and refined grains make up a (conservative) 50 percent of caloric intake! Both sugar and refined grains wreak havoc with health in myriad ways. We'll discuss sugar's detriments in chapter 5.

Antibiotics and other drugs. The overuse of certain medicines—such as antibiotics and steroids, both in our children and in the animal foods they eat—can lead to imbalances in the endocrine system, the immune system, and in gut bacteria, all of which negatively affect the whole body. Keeping immunity strong will create less need for such drugs, and choosing higher-quality animal foods will also reduce exposure to them.

Processed foods. Processed foods are devitalized and fake, containing multiple harmful and damaging man-made ingredients, from growth hormone to rancid fats to genetically engineered components. These kinds of foods deplete the body of precious nutrient stores and give nothing back but calories and toxins. They are also difficult to digest and can lead to gut problems, food allergies, and autoimmune conditions.

Wrong macronutrient ratios at meals. When babies and children are fed typical "kid-food" diets, often they become

A house that is spacious and strongly built will serve as a pleasant home for many, many years, even if the occupants are less than conscientious about the upkeep. And if such a house falls into disrepair it can be brought back to good condition with the proper attention. But a house that is poorly built may never be comfortable and will require constant maintenance just to keep it from falling down.

Most children growing up today live in the latter type of house. Throughout life, in order to be healthy, such individuals will need to pay very careful attention to their diets at all times. Their houses will likely be constantly springing leaks—allergies, digestive problems, fatigue, behavior abnormalities, etc.

reliant on carbohydrates and don't get adequate healthy fats and protein. The Standard American Diet is at least two-thirds carbohydrate based. Even the new USDA MyPlate portions are approximately three-quarters fruits, veggies, and grains—all of which are carbohydrates. SADly, much of modern carbohydrate intake is sugar and refined grain, with very little nutrition to offer. The false sense that sufficient calories alone will enable proper growth and development has excused the consistently poor food quality fed to babies and children for too long. (We cover carbs in chapters 5 and 6.)

Super Nutrition Builds Super Health for Your Baby

The goal of our Super Nutrition Baby Feeding Program is to empower you to take your baby's health destiny into your own hands. By doing this, you will gain the skills to strengthen and protect your baby, maximizing both her mental and physical health potential and reducing her chances of developing 3C conditions. What you feed your baby now will impact both her immediate and lifelong health.

In the foreword of the book *Healing Our Children*, Sally Fallon Morell, author, researcher, traditional-foods advocate, and founder and president of the Weston A. Price Foundation, provides the wonderful example of how fortifying your child's body is analogous to building a house. (See opposite page.)

Considering the well-known story of the Three Little Pigs, we ask: What kind of "house" are you building for your child? Straw-and-twig houses are easiest to blow over—

built with too few Allies and allowing an overabundance of Enemy influences and attacks (a forest full of wolves). However, Super Nutrition ensures that you'll build the strongest house possible for your baby (a sturdy brick house), optimizing the support of children's health Allies while minimizing exposure to Enemies.

The Pillars of Super Nutrition

We've built our Super Nutrition Baby Feeding Program on the foundation of protective nutrition. On this foundation stand four pillars, which are scientifically and clinically sound. We have incorporated medical research, the findings of several experts, scientific evidence, and our own clinical experience to focus on those factors that most influence children's health when it comes to 3C conditions. To prevent the 3Cs from taking hold, you must carefully select and prepare your baby's foods to be the most *digestible, pure, immune bolstering, and nutrient worthy*. We'll discuss in detail what these foods are and how to do this in the coming chapters, but first we'll explain the four pillars of Super Nutrition.

PILLAR #1: DIGESTIBILITY. FACILITATE DIGESTION AND SUPPORT INTESTINAL HEALTH.

You can make digestion easier for your baby if you provide her with the right foods (see chapter 2). Acknowledging that an infant's digestive system is different than that of an older child or adult is important in determining when you can introduce certain foods. How you prepare the food also makes a significant difference in digestibility. We will guide you in choosing and making easy-to-digest foods for your baby at each stage.

Natasha Campbell-McBride, M.D., focuses on the neuro-logic- and psychiatric-based 3Cs (autism, depression, ADD, etc.) in her book *Gut and Psychology Syndrome (GAPS)*. Dr. Campbell-McBride, a neurologist, nutrition expert, and autism specialist, suggests that since the digestive system impacts immunity, availability of nutrients, protection from toxins, and detoxification of toxins, it directly affects the health and functioning of the brain.

But there's more to it and, writes Dr. Campbell-McBride, "the gut-brain connection is something . . . many modern doctors do not understand." There's actually a "second brain" in the gut; though it doesn't "think" con-scious thoughts, it *does* affect behavior. It is not only the master of digestion, but the gut also conveys massive quantities of information to the brain. In addition to impacting nutritional status and immunity, intestinal health also influences mood, behavior, mental health, and emotion.

Digestible foods are those that:

▸ Have had their digestive irritants neutralized (soaked, sprouted, or leavened)

▸ Are predigested (fermented or cultured)

▸ Contain enzymes (as in raw animal foods, tropical fruits, and fermented or cultured foods)

PILLAR #2: PURITY. REDUCE TOXIC EXPOSURE AND IMPROVE DETOXIFICATION CAPABILITIES.

Our program will suggest foods that are least processed and least toxic. Avoiding even a few ingredients will go a long way in reducing the toxic burden your child carries. *Purity* is a criterion we hope you'll begin to apply to feed-ing choices for your baby.

In light of the toxic reality babies face today (see chapter 3), detoxification is crucial. Luckily, your baby has built-in systems for detoxification—based on natural mechanisms that are designed to protect her. Unfortunately, this detoxi-fication ability is often decreased due to nutrient deficien-cies and toxins that can further block detoxification path-ways. Consequently, optimizing nutrition and reducing toxin exposure are critical to detoxification and thus, good health and optimal development.

Ideally, pure foods meet the following criteria:

▸ No additives, synthetic nutrient "fortification," preser-vatives, or other chemical additives

▸ No artificial sweeteners, colorings, or flavorings

▸ Organic—sustainably grown in nutrient-rich soils, with-out the use of chemical pesticides

▸ From animals that have eaten their natural diet (pas-ture fed)

▸ No growth hormone, antibiotics, or other drugs given to farm animals

▸ In whole form—not refined, isolated, or concentrated

▸ Minimally processed

▸ Not genetically modified

PILLAR #3: IMMUNE BOOSTING. STRENGTHEN AND SUPPORT IMMUNITY.

You can foster a stronger immune system through nutrient-rich feeding, proper digestion, and purposeful microbial exposure (more in chapter 4). In particular, healthy bacterial exposure and colonization is critical to a healthy body and strong immune system.

Getting or being sick with viral or bacterial infections can cause more than just the uncomfortable symptoms. Infections—when they take root—excessively burden the body, cause inflammation, and use up priceless nutrients and enzymes, as the body works to regain a healthy balance. The proper functioning of your baby's immune system is very important to the big picture of health because *staying healthy is easier on the body than getting health back once infection sets in.*

Surprisingly, the best way to prevent infection isn't to avoid microbes. It is actually to fortify the immune system from within. Since the vast majority of microbes are *good*—and those few that *could* make us sick don't always do so when we're exposed to them—it's the state of our body's health and immune capabilities that determine whether we will actually get sick.

Immune-boosting foods are those that:
▸ Support the immune system with critical nutrients
▸ Supply living immune cells (as in mom's milk and raw mammalian milk)
▸ Provide probiotics
▸ Supply enzymes

PILLAR #4: NUTRIENT WORTH. PROVIDE OPTIMALLY NOURISHING FOODS.

Foods that are most nutritious are not commonly found in the Standard American Diet. Our program will educate you about what makes a food truly nourishing (see chapter 6). Part of this pillar also includes avoiding foods that rob your baby of nutrients or contain nutrient blockers (see chapter 5). *Nutrient worth* is an important way to judge foods— they should be "worthy" of supporting your baby's growth and development.

Focusing on nutrient-rich foods is worthwhile because they have been shown via extensive research to build healthy, robust babies. Revolutionary nutrition researcher and dentist Weston A. Price, D.D.S., studied health among cultures across the six inhabited continents of the globe during the 1920s and 1930s. He used saliva, food samples, observation, medical and dental examinations, interviews, skeletal-remains studies, and photographic evidence to do his research. He reported his findings in his book *Nutrition and Physical Degeneration*, which has remained a seminal work on nutrition and health.

Dr. Price conducted his studies at a unique time in history, when many primitive stocks of people had yet to be touched by modern industry. He specifically chose peoples who were living and eating off their land as they had for thousands of years. At this time, he was also witness to the building of roads, the coming of boats, and the arrival of missionaries who brought "industrialized" foods such as jellies, jams, canned meats, and white flour. In his studies that spanned two decades, he saw that the generation eating "modern" foods got sick far more than the same genetic stock not eating modern foods and also gave birth to unhealthy babies! He later documented that a return to the traditional-foods diet would restore their health.

Dr. Price found that lack of proper nutrition was *causal* in physical degeneration and most chronic diseases. He concluded that optimal nutrition was key to both physical *re*generation and the prevention of degenerative disease.

Foods with high nutrient worth are those that:

▸ Are nutrient dense, containing a rich amount of nutrients per calorie

▸ Do not contain antinutrients that block mineral absorption

▸ Do not contain sugars or refined salt

These four pillars of Super Nutrition have guided each and every recommendation in this book. By focusing on them, you can expect your baby to have the best overall health on many levels—including but not limited to strong immune system functioning, emotional control, focus, dental health and orthodontic positioning, metabolic functioning, and countless other facets of well-being. With Super Nutrition, you will be helping your baby to become the smartest, happiest, and healthiest she can possibly be.

Got Raw? When It Comes to Milk, Fresh Is Best!

Throughout all of our recommendations for healthy baby feeding—from mom's nursing diet and homemade formula to weaning beverages and first foods—we'll be suggesting fresh, raw milk. No doubt, this raises a lot of questions.

Raw milk is *not pasteurized* milk; it is fresh and in its natural state. Realistically, raw milk should just be called "milk" and pasteurized milk should be called "processed milk." Raw milk is better because it is fresh, intact, and unadulterated. In this state, it is a *healing* food that is meant to sustain life and nourish those who consume it. Fresh milk confers nutritional, digestive, and immune benefits. Fresh, raw dairy from cows is remarkably similar to fresh raw milk from humans.

Raw, fresh milk from a trusted, clean dairy comes from cows that are allowed to graze on green pastures in sunlight and fresh air. Raw, fresh milk cows are also *not* given drugs, growth hormone, and antibiotics, so raw milk does not contain toxins. Furthermore, raw milk's transit time from cow to consumer is very short, making the milk very fresh when you consume it.

Milk in this pure state, from such nourished cows, upholds all four pillars of Super Nutrition. Raw milk is worth getting from the farm for four main reasons:

1. With a complete suite of enzymes, the milk aids digestion and even digests itself.
2. Raw milk is free of toxins, such as drugs, vaccinations, synthetic nutrients, and pesticides.
3. Raw milk is an immune booster.
4. Raw milk is a healing, Super POWER food, rich in vitamins and very rich in absorbable minerals.

Pasteurization is processing of milk with high heat to kill bacteria and other pathogens that might have contaminated the milk. These bacteria don't naturally occur in the milk, but rather can contaminate it during collection, further processing, and storage. Back in the early 1900s, when cleanliness wasn't a priority, city-milk cows (not on pasture) were kept in filth and fed poorly, and milk containers were reused and not washed. These sick cows and deplorable conditions led to rampant contamination of milk, which made many people sick. Pasteurization was developed to sterilize *this* kind of milk.

Yet the conventional dairies of the modern day aren't much better than those early city dairies. Their cows are fed unnatural diets and kept in dirty, cramped conditions, which makes pasteurization necessary. But unfortunately, pasteurization doesn't ensure the milk is safe. *Pasteurized milk can easily be contaminated after sterilization (pasteurization), just like your hands can get dirty after you've washed them.*

On the contrary, raw-milk farms are very different from modern operations and resemble the ideal farm from days of old. Grazing cows have healthier guts and healthy bacteria growing within. Before milking, the cows' teats are cleaned with iodine to kill potential bacteria, and the milk is collected into a sterile stainless container and immediately refrigerated. Typically, from milking to consumers' refrigerator takes only 24 to 48 hours. With such minimal storage, no processing, and limited transportation, there is very little chance for raw milk to be exposed to contaminants. But even if it were somehow contaminated, raw milk keeps itself healthy. Its living immune factors and enzyme-based pathogen killers can stop the bad bugs just like mom's milk does. It's these living components in milk—hormones, enzymes, heat sensitive nutrients, and probiotics—that are damaged, denatured, or rendered inactive after pasteurization and homogenization. This processing renders a health food into one that is allergenic and irritating to the immune system.

On the contrary, raw milk is protective. In September 2011, Reuters Health reported on a study published in the *Journal of Allergy and Clinical Immunology,* announcing: "Kids who drink raw milk have less asthma, allergies." The GABRIELA study of more than 8,000 children showed that raw milk consumption was inversely related to asthma, atopy (allergies), and hay fever! Reuters stated that according to this large study, "Children who drink raw milk are less likely to develop asthma and allergies than those who stick to the … pasteurized version." In fact, raw-milk drinkers had a *41 percent reduction* in chances of developing asthma compared to store-bought or boiled milk drinkers. Their chances of developing hay fever were reduced *by half* if they drank raw milk. This corroborates earlier studies showing that "farm milk" is protective against such 3C conditions and their symptoms. Whether due to the unadulterated whey proteins in raw milk or its immune-boosting components, helpful hormones, enzymes, or the wholesome suite of vitamins and absorbable minerals—we aren't quite sure. We do know that these constituents are destroyed or damaged in pasteurized milk, so it doesn't have these coveted positive effects. Quite clearly—and scientifically shown—raw milk (and *not pasteurized*) has potent protective benefits for children against 3C conditions!

Raw milk from a clean, trusted dairy is not only safe, it is one of the *best* elements in your child's diet or yours if you're a nursing mom. Visit www.realmilk.com to find fresh-milk dairies near you. In some states, raw milk is available for purchase in grocery stores. In many, though, you're required to join a "cow-share" program directly with the farm. Basically, this means you pay for the care and feeding of your cow, and you're entitled to the dairy products of that cow.

A FURTHER Q&A ON RAW MILK

Q: Isn't there bacteria in raw, unpasteurized milk?

A: Milk itself—from any mammal—is not inherently infected with pathogens. Mammals' milk is designed to nourish infants who have immature immune systems, so if milk naturally contained pathogens, babies would die, and species wouldn't survive. Milk can become contaminated with bacteria if cleanliness measures are not taken or if the cows providing the milk are not healthy. Thus it is critical to obtain raw milk from the highest-quality farm with the healthiest of animals.

Q: Isn't pasteurized milk safer to buy than raw milk?

A: Raw milk is a surprisingly safe food compared not only to pasteurized milk, but also all foods. After statistical analysis relating to the four most common pathogens and foodborne illness they cause, Ted Beals, M.S, M.D., reports that *less than* 42 cases of the annual 1,937,561 cases of food-borne illnesses are attributable to raw milk consumption. That means that 1,937,519 cases are caused by foods *other* than raw milk. Relatively speaking, you're very safe drinking raw milk! *Pasteurization offers a false sense of security*. Pasteurized milk can and does get contaminated and cause food-borne illness. According to William Campbell Douglass II, M.D., author of *The Raw Truth about Milk*, "Over the past few decades, outbreaks due to pasteurized milk have led to well over 200,000 cases of food poisoning and over 600 deaths." *Pasteurization does absolutely nothing to protect the milk from becoming contaminated* after *it is pasteurized*. At one of the largest raw milk farms in California, a 10-year study showed *no cases* of their raw milk causing illness.

Q: Why not go "dairy free"?

A: In terms of going dairy free, we warn you: Don't throw the baby out with the bathwater. Real milk is the richest source of minerals and several other nutrients available to us in our modern, nutrient-depleted diet. With its immune-supporting factors, enzymes, vitamins, and probiotics, it might well be the healthiest element of your (or your child's) diet. Sweet-tasting fresh milk and butter, as well as cheese and more-tart yogurt and kefir, can absolutely do a body good and be part of Super Nutrition—they are *healing* foods. Raw milk is the easiest way to get amazing nutrition into your child. If you do nothing else except provide raw dairy, you'll be doing a great favor to your children.

Q: What if raw milk were to get contaminated? Wouldn't it make me sick?

A: As with any food—from peanut butter to spinach—contamination with bacteria has the possibility of making people sick. However, studies show that raw milk can be exposed to *Salmonella, Listeria, and E. coli* and due to its enzymes and living immune cells, can completely destroy or stop the pathogens from growing! The same bugs dropped in pasteurized milk, which is sterile and devoid of immune protectors, would have nothing to stop them from proliferating and would completely contaminate the milk, which is why there are so many cases of foodborne illness from pasteurized milk. *Further, government figures show that people are 35,000 times more like to contract food-borne illness from other foods than they are from raw milk.* For more information visit: http://westonaprice.org/press/government-data-proves-raw-milk-safe.

Super Nutrition Food Categories

To make Super Nutrition simpler to implement, we've created Super Nutrition food categories to easily illustrate which foods are most important to avoid and which are most critical in your baby's diet. We hope this will help you make decisions when you procure your baby's food.

We've grouped foods in accordance with the four pillars and categorized them as either CRAP, OKAY, PURE, or Super POWER foods. We'll refer to these categories throughout the remaining chapters as a helpful tool for you in meal planning, purchasing, and preparation. The handy acronyms will help you understand why each of the foods belongs in the category where we have slated it and will help you identify food quality as you feed your baby. Eventually you'll come to recognize whether a certain food incorporates elements of Super Nutrition.

CRAP FOODS

Stated purposefully in such a vulgar way, CRAP foods contribute to the toxic burden your baby must carry. They do not provide proper nutrition and detract from the nutrients your baby needs for growth, development, detoxification, and immunity. Refer to the acronym CRAP to help you remember why you want to eliminate, or at least minimize, these foods in your baby's diet.

▸ **CRAP**
Chemical
Removes body's nutrients
Addictive
Processed

Foods that are in the CRAP category do not meet any of the criteria within the pillars of Super Nutrition: They are not digestible, they are not pure, they are not immune boosting, and they are not nutrient worthy. Most processed foods fall into this category.

Counter to being protective, CRAP foods are most often *harmful*. When you feed them to your child, not only are you *not* supporting proper health, growth, or development—you are likely hindering these processes, adding to your baby's toxic burden and reducing nutrient abilities. We realize that all children will have some CRAP foods, but we also want to be sure you understand how important it is to reduce them as much as possible. CRAP foods include the following:

▸ Fast food and prepackaged meals (especially microwavable)
▸ Foods made with white flour (crackers, pretzels, bagels, and bread)
▸ Most school lunches
▸ Margarine
▸ Vegetable oils (cottonseed, corn, soy, and canola)
▸ Cereal
▸ Candy and other white-sugar-containing foods
▸ Cookies, snack bars, cereal bars, and protein bars
▸ Nonorganic lunch meat
▸ Soda pop and store-bought juice
▸ Most soy products, including soy formula
▸ Nonorganic, low-fat, pasteurized dairy
▸ Organic ultrapasteurized dairy
▸ Genetically modified organisms/foods (GMOs) (soy, corn, canola, beet sugar, high fructose corn syrup, and cottonseed)
▸ Refined white salt

OKAY FOODS

While these foods aren't the very best available, they are often part of the Standard American Diet. They are convenient, easy to come by, inexpensive, and found in most grocery stores. Truthfully, it is hard to have a diet that doesn't include OKAY foods. While a diet of only OKAY foods won't be adequate to provide Super Nutrition, they can be okay as *part* of a healthier diet. If your baby's diet is made up of some OKAY foods, some PURE foods, and some Super POWER foods, you will be doing very well by her.

> ▸ **OKAY**
> ▸ **O**rdinary
> ▸ **K**nockoffs of real food
> ▸ **A**dequate, not optimal
> ▸ **Y**ield subpar health if fed exclusively

Some of the foods that we list as OKAY you might not have categorized here. Better choices could be made that would provide superior nutrition and health support. OKAY foods include the following:

▸ Unsoaked and unsprouted whole grains and legumes
▸ Unsoaked and unsprouted nuts and seeds
▸ Dried fruits
▸ Grocery-store eggs
▸ All-natural and organic grain-fed meat
▸ Farmed fish
▸ Pasteurized (not ultrapasteurized), organic, full-fat dairy products
▸ Fresh-squeezed juice
▸ Nonorganic vegetables
▸ Nonorganic fruit
▸ Nut butters
▸ Organic, nitrite-free lunch meat

▸ Fermented non-GMO soy
▸ Whole-foods sweeteners (raw honey, Rapadura, coconut palm sugar, etc.)

PURE FOODS

These foods are clean, digestible, and offer improved nutrient richness. They are important to incorporate into your child's diet as much as possible, as they support the serious nutrient needs of the body, aiding in cognitive, neurological, immune, and physical development.

> ▸ **PURE**
> ▸ **P**asture based
> ▸ **U**nadulterated
> ▸ **R**ich in nutrients
> ▸ **E**nzyme containing

In a perfect world, the ideal diet for your child would consist of only PURE and Super POWER foods. Yet more realistically, if we consume some OKAY foods but we are sure to also include Super POWER foods and rely mostly on PURE foods for our baby's nutrition, we'll far exceed "average" and improve the 3C disease statistics that come with average baby feeding. PURE foods include the following:

▸ Soaked or sprouted whole grains and legumes
▸ Soaked or sprouted nuts and seeds
▸ Organic, local, seasonal, fruits and vegetables
▸ Organic tropical fruits
▸ Eggs from free-range chickens eating an omega-3 enriched diet
▸ Pastured/grass-fed meats, poultry, and pork
▸ Wild-caught fish and seafood
▸ Unrefined, cold-pressed oils (olive oil) and tropical fats (coconut and palm)
▸ Low-temp (VAT) pasteurized, organic, grass-fed, nonhomogenized dairy products

Johnny Davies' First Two Years

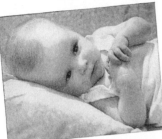

John at 3 months weighs 12 pounds, 7 ounces. He is one of a group of babies in Westfield, N. J., whose growth and development are being studied under scientific supervision. Cereal has just come into Johnny's life—Clapp's Strained Baby Cereal.

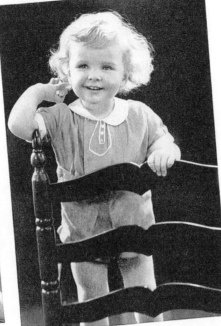

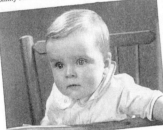

John at 7 months has been gradually introduced to all the Clapp soups, vegetables and fruits. Rich in vitamins and minerals, conserved by quick pressure-cooking, these foods are real bodybuilders—as Johnny's chart shows. He weighs 15 pounds, 8 ounces, and sat alone at 6½ months.

John at 22 months weighs 31 pounds and has the hearty appetite for all the "protective" foods which is characteristic of Clapp-fed children. For Clapp's Foods really do taste better—they're delicious in flavor and delicately seasoned. And they have the texture that specialists recommend—smoothly strained, but not too liquid.

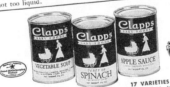

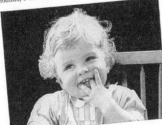

John at 12 months is a perfect picture of a sturdy year-old baby. Clapp's Strained Foods have continued to play an important role in his diet. He weighs 22 pounds, 3 ounces, has been creeping for almost 3 months, and can stand without support.

17 VARIETIES

Soups: Baby Soup (Strained), Baby Soup (Unstrained), Vegetable Soup, Beef Broth, Liver Soup.
Vegetables: Tomatoes, Asparagus, Spinach, Peas, Beets, Carrots, Green Beans, Mixed Greens.
Fruits: Apricots, Prunes, Apple Sauce.
Cereal: Baby Cereal.

FREE BOOKLET—"12 Babies Tell Their Own Story," a fascinating photo-history of the first year in the lives of a dozen Clapp-fed babies. Valuable feeding information, charts and special baby recipes. Use the Congratulations reply card or write to:

CLAPP'S STRAINED BABY FOODS
777 Mount Read Blvd., Rochester, N. Y.

SUPER POWER FOODS

These foods are digestible, pure, immune boosting, and nutrient worthy—and as a result, they can protect and even regenerate and restore health. They are absolutely the "superheroes" of the diet, found by researchers, nutritionists, historians, and anthropologists to be traditionally honored as "sacred" foods.

▶ **POWER**
- ▶ **P**rotective
- ▶ **O**ptimal nutrition
- ▶ **W**isdom of the ancients
- ▶ **E**nriching
- ▶ **R**egenerating

Super POWER foods have qualities most other foods don't:
- ▶ Complete, whole, real, natural foods
- ▶ Nutrient dense and uniquely able to heal
- ▶ Part of traditional wisdom and used by ancient cultures for healing
- ▶ Free of toxins
- ▶ Packed with a wide array of antioxidants, vitamins, and minerals
- ▶ Supply inflammation fighters
- ▶ Often a source of the all-important, fat-soluble mineral activators
- ▶ Many also contain probiotics and enzymes

What can Super POWER foods do that other foods can't? They are heavy-hitting, healing foods. They are literally the "strongest" against pre-existing problems and act as preventive measures in the diet. Due to their super nutrition, they are the best to support the body, to build the brain, bolster gut integrity, heal tooth decay, grow optimally healthy babies during pregnancy and after, and fortify mom's milk to enable ideal development for babies during nursing. Few foods have this kind of résumé.

We give much credit to researchers and nutrition pioneers who've studied preindustrialized peoples to understand their natural and traditional eating habits. It is from such research, like that of Dr. Price, that we've learned what should be held sacred in our diets. Science has corroborated that these sacred foods are the most nutrient dense available and therefore confer the most health benefits.

Dr. Price's research particularly highlights the importance of fat-soluble activators, which allow minerals to be used in the body. Fat-soluble activators are the mortar, and minerals are the bricks, of the healthy house you're building for your baby; they need each other to work effectively. Many of our Super POWER foods are classified as such because they contain these mineral-activating vitamins (A, D3, and K2). Minerals are critical to health, and as Dr. Price warned, "It is possible to *starve for minerals* that are abundant in the foods eaten *because they cannot be utilized without an adequate quantity of the fat-soluble activators*." Super POWER foods include the following:
- ▶ Liver and other organ meats from pastured, organically raised animals
- ▶ Cod liver oil and high-vitamin butter oil

- Raw, grass-fed, organic dairy and cultured dairy
- Pasture-fed animal fats and raw butter from grass-fed cows
- Bone marrow
- Mineral-rich bone-based soup stock
- Eggs from organic, free-range poultry
- Oily, whole seafood (e.g., sardines) and shellfish from clean sources
- Fish roe
- Probiotic-rich condiments (chutney, salsa, sauerkraut)
- Lacto-fermented beverages (yogurt, gingerale, kombucha, kefir)
- Celtic sea salt and Himalayan sea salt

At first you might think your child won't like these foods. Yet parents whom we've seen in our practice are often surprised to find that their babies *love* them.

PUTTING IT ALL TOGETHER

We know that some of the foods we recommend will seem strange to your modern tastes and habits. But keep in mind that they are the most nutrient-dense foods on Earth; for almost all of human history, they've been the source of nourishment for adults and children alike. If you were told that you could improve the likelihood that your child would seldom get sick, thrive developmentally, avoid a whole host of physical and psychological diseases now and in her future, and improve the health of future generations, wouldn't you jump at the chance? Well, we're telling you that it is possible, and we'll explain how feeding your child better can make all the difference.

Mom to Mom / Many of the items that we recommend for Super Nutrition must be of the highest quality, such as liver, lard, coconut milk, and fish roe. Unfortunately, these are not often found at your local grocery store; thus, online shopping is incredibly helpful. Keep two lists throughout the month—a shopping list and an online ordering list. Once a month, place your online orders. Try visiting http://blog.grasslandbeef.com/super-nutrition-for-babies-0/ as a source of pastured, organic meats and organ meats, game, wild caught seafood and more.

Though you might be motivated to provide a 100 percent Super POWER diet, realistically we expect that your child will be fed a diet made up of a mixture of CRAP, OKAY, PURE, and some Super POWER foods. We live in a busy, modern, convenience-driven world with peculiar social expectations around food and feeding, which don't always nicely accommodate traditional foods (such as those important for Super Nutrition). But even just reducing CRAP foods, increasing PURE foods, and offering some Super POWER foods when you can will significantly contribute to your child's health. This book offers you a better way to feed your baby than what social standards currently dictate. By taking the road less traveled, you'll be guiding your baby to a better health destiny than where she'd otherwise end up if she were to eat as "everyone else" does.

Super Nutrition Food Categories

▶ CRAP foods

Chemical
Removes body's nutrients
Addictive
Processed (not natural)

- White flour–based foods: cereal, crackers, pretzels, breads, bagels
- White sugar: candy, candy bars, baked goods
- Refined white salt
- Nonorganic, low-fat, pasteurized dairy; any ultrapasteurized dairy (even organic)
- Additives, colorings, preservatives, MSG, GMO, artificial sweeteners
- Vegetable oils: corn, cottonseed, soy, canola oil; margarine
- Fast food, highly processed meats, most school lunches
- Store-bought juice, soda pop
- Most soy products (including soy formula)

▶ OKAY foods

Ordinary
Knockoffs of real food
Adequate, not optimal
Yield subpar health

- All-natural and organic meat from grain-fed animals
- Unsoaked and unsprouted whole grains and legumes
- Grocery store eggs
- Nonorganic fruits and vegetables
- Unsoaked and unsprouted nuts, seeds, and nut butters
- Farmed fish and seafood
- Whole-foods sweeteners (e.g., raw honey, Rapadura)
- Fresh-squeezed, fresh juices with veggies and fruit
- Fermented non-GMO soy (miso, natto, tempeh)
- Organic, full-fat pasteurized dairy
- Dried fruits
- Organic, nitrite-free lunch meat

▶ PURE foods

Pasture based
Unadulterated
Rich in nutrients
Enzyme containing

- Organic, local, seasonal fruits and veggies
- Organic tropical fruits
- Vat-pasteurized, nonhomogenized, organic, grass-fed dairy
- Grass-fed meats, poultry, and pork
- Sea vegetables (kelp, nori, spirulina)
- Wild-caught fish and seafood
- Soaked or sprouted nuts and seeds
- Organic free-range eggs from chickens fed an omega-3 enriched diet
- Sprouted or soaked whole grains and legumes
- Unrefined cold-pressed oils (e.g., olive oil) and tropical fats (e.g., coconut and palm)

▶ POWER foods

Protective
Optimal nutrition
Wisdom of the ancients
Enriching
Regenerating

- Liver and other organ meats from pastured, organically raised animals
- Lacto-fermented drinks (e.g., kombucha, kefir)
- Organic farm-fresh, pasture-raised eggs
- Probiotic-rich foods (e.g., raw dairy, yogurt, kefir, sauerkraut, kimchi, and other lacto-fermented foods)
- Pasture-fed animal fats such as raw butter
- Oily, whole seafood (e.g., sardines) and shellfish
- Mineral-rich bone-based soup stock
- Raw, whole-fat, grass-fed dairy
- Fish roe
- Bone marrow
- Celtic sea salt or Himalayan sea salt
- Cod liver oil and high-vitamin butter oil

Your Baby's Health Is in Your Hands

Literally, as it's in this book! Even if you follow just some of our recommendations, you will improve your child's odds for achieving and maintaining optimal wellness. We realize our suggestions are often off the beaten path and take significantly more effort than just opening a jar or reheating in the microwave. We know what we're asking of you is significant—in terms of time and effort; we know this firsthand because we've been there as mothers as well as practitioners and have guided countless patients through this process. We also know what is at stake if you do not make the extra effort in feeding your baby following Super Nutrition style; we have worked even harder to recover health in our own children and in our patients who've fallen victim to 3Cs because a traditional-foods diet was not followed.

This book will provide you with what you need to know; the more closely you incorporate Super Nutrition feeding practices, the more *protected* your child will be. Of course the converse is also true: The more you compromise, or fall into "normal" ways that kids are typically fed (albeit easier and more convenient), the more you will allow the Enemies to challenge your child's health.

Put Super Nutrition in place by following our guidelines and recommendations. You will create the strongest foundation for your baby, maximizing her current and long-term health. We know that as a parent, you wouldn't want it any other way for your baby.

In the following chapters, we'll walk you through the ages and stages you'll cherish as your baby grows. Along the way, we'll guide you and educate you about development, nutritional needs, and the best way to nourish your baby, supplying "Allied" reinforcements to keep her safe from "Enemies" in her diet and environment. We are so happy that this imperative book has reached you—so that you can follow the appropriate guidelines toward optimal health for your darling baby.

From Fake Flakes to Real Food

Meeting Nutrient Needs with First Foods

6 to 8 Months

It's so exciting to start feeding your baby first foods. Weeks in advance, many parents prepare: stocking up on bibs, spoons, and little bowls. It *is* fun. Many parents are also eager for their babies to try new foods as soon as they're able. Maybe you're just as eager. But we urge you not to rush it. It's important that your baby is ready—developmentally, physically, and digestively—before you begin feeding him first foods. By waiting until he's ready, you'll be facilitating digestion and intestinal health, which together comprise the first pillar (digestibility) of Super Nutrition.

Developing Digestion

If you feed your baby solid foods before he can digest them, he won't benefit from their nutrients. In the early months of life, your baby cannot digest solid foods because his pancreas doesn't make many of its own digestive enzymes. Also, he is still building up friendly flora (probiotics) along his intestinal wall, which will eventually make digestive enzymes too. Without his own digestive enzymes and digestion-aiding beneficial bacteria, he relies on mom's milk (or formula) as a source of "predigested" food.

Enzymes are the "keys" that unlock the bonds in food molecules, allowing them to be broken down into their tiniest building blocks (digestion). It is the building blocks that are usable by his body for growth, biochemical processes, and energy.

For healthy function, proteins need to be digested all the way down to their building blocks (called amino acids); carbohydrates into single sugars (glucose); and fats into individual fatty acids. If foods aren't fully digested into their building blocks, they simply aren't useful. Even worse, undigested foods can cause health troubles.

Risks of undigested foods include food allergies, digestive distress, autoimmune conditions (like celiac disease), toxic overload, overstimulation of the immune system, nutrient deficiencies, inflammation, cognitive complications resulting from neurotoxicity, and other health problems.

Critical Nutrients at 6 Months

While your baby's digestive system won't be fully "grown up" until at least 2 years of age, at around 6 months, he'll have some very particular nutrient needs that are best met by introducing solid foods. Also, your baby's accelerated growth means that his caloric intake needs are growing, too. He needs to supplement mom's milk or formula because these liquids alone no longer provide him with enough energy to sustain his rapidly growing body.

Avoiding Food Allergies

Food allergies come from undigested protein and "open," or "leaky," gut walls. In the early months, your baby has openings in his intestinal lining—a normal state called "open" gut. This allows good antibodies from mom's milk to pass through his gut wall easily into his bloodstream, where they can protect him.

However, if foods are introduced while the gut is leaky, undigested foods can get into the bloodstream through the openings. When the immune system sees whole or only partially digested proteins, it views them as foreign invaders and attacks. The food's identity is put into the immune memory bank, so the next time that undigested food makes it into the bloodstream, the immune system will attack again. This is a food allergy. Common symptoms of food allergies are colic, abdominal distention, gas, spitting up, rash/eczema/hives, congestion, swollen mouth, cough, and/or difficulty breathing.

This 1948 ad for Swift's Strained Meats states, during "actual feeding tests," doctors felt that "meat-fed babies were in *better physical condition generally*!" The ad notes "All medical statements made in this advertisement are accepted by the . . . American Medical Association." With Swift's, your baby "gets to know the distinctive flavor of six tempting meats he will eat all his life: beef, lamb, pork, veal, liver, and heart." Unlike a few generations ago, many babies today never taste lamb, liver, or heart—and certainly do not eat them throughout life; yet these special meats offer superior nutrition.

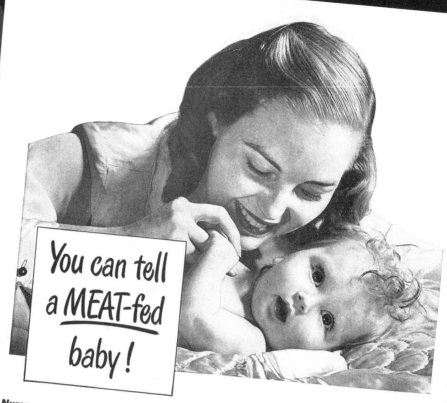

You can tell a <u>MEAT</u>-fed baby!

Nurses report: babies on Swift's Strained Meats were more satisfied . . . slept better at night!

What a big difference meat makes to a little baby! During actual feeding tests with bottle-fed infants, nurses reported that babies who received Swift's Strained Meats in their formulas were "more satisfied and slept better at night"† than babies who received no meat. Doctors felt that meat-fed babies were in *better physical condition generally!* They had good red blood, too—*higher* hemoglobin level and *better* blood value! Now, with these specially prepared Swift's Strained Meats, it's easy to give your own baby this head start on health!*

Meat — to grow on!

Swift's Strained Meats provide complete high-quality proteins—the kind baby needs for sound, sturdy growth

SWIFT & COMPANY •

—B vitamins plus blood building iron which helps prevent anemia. Swift's Strained Meats are 100% meat, not mixtures. Because you feed them separately, you help baby form good eating habits. He gets to know the distinctive flavor of six tempting meats he will be eating all his life: beef, lamb, pork, veal, liver and heart. Stock up now on Swift's Strained and Swift's Diced Meats at your neighborhood food store.

†*Meat in the Diet of Young Infants—Ruth M. Leverton, Ph.D. and George Clark, M.D. Journal of the American Medical Association J.A.M.A., 134: 1215, August 9, 1947)*

*ASK YOUR DOCTOR *when to start and the amount of Swift's Strained Meats to feed. You'll be surprised at how much meat a fast-growing baby can eat!*

CHICAGO 9, ILLINOIS

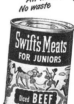

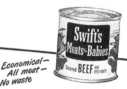

Economical— All meat— No waste

All nutritional statements made in this advertisement are accepted by the Council on Foods and Nutrition of the American Medical Association.

Swift's Diced Meats for Juniors
Chopped—tender and juicy. (Confidentially, the whole family will go for these meats!)

SWIFT...*foremost name in meats* ...*<u>first</u> with 100% Meats for Babies*

SWIFT QUALITY FOODS

JULY, 1948

7

Babies accumulate plenty of iron and zinc while in utero, but by 6 months old, much of these stores have been used up. Mom's milk offers very absorbable iron and zinc, but typically not enough to meet the monumental nutrient demands of rapid growth between 6 and 12 months.

Ironclad blood and brain are best. Without iron, babies' brains are hit hard. They need iron for normal neurologic development. In babies who don't get enough, doctors find irreversible cognitive and motor damage. *The scariest part is that even if iron is replenished, the damage may be irreversible.* Iron deficiency is tragically common; your best course of action is to include foods rich in absorbable iron—that is, animal foods—on a regular basis. Note that while pediatricians check for anemia through bloodwork, studies show damage to the brain can occur *before* low iron shows up on such tests.

Zinc is the link for immunity, growth, and learning. Zinc contributes to the health of your baby's immune system, intestinal mucosal lining, and skin and influences physical activity, growth, and cognitive development. If levels of zinc are too low, growth will slow, diarrheal disease can be more common, immune function will be impaired, and eczema may develop.

According to a study in the *American Journal of Clinical Nutrition*, zinc stimulates healthier bones, and low zinc is shown to stunt growth. Animal foods have the highest zinc content in the most absorbable form; therefore, it is no surprise that vegan children, especially boys, tend to be shorter. In fact, according to current research, having enough zinc from birth through age 5 can metabolically "program" your child's height.

Higher zinc levels might also lead to improved cognitive development. In a randomized, controlled study, cited by the *Journal of Pediatric Gastroenterology and Nutrition*, researchers compared introducing meat or iron-fortified cereal for exclusively breast-fed infants. What were the results? The meat-fed infants had substantially higher zinc levels than did cereal-fed infants, had a higher rate of brain growth, and demonstrated likely trends "toward other developmental advantages."

Watch for blockers. Some foods contain iron and zinc *blockers,* which decrease the availability of these minerals. Blocker-containing foods include soy, grains, legumes, tea, and antacids.

Don't rely on plant or "fortified" foods. "Fortified" foods and plant sources have a form of iron called *nonheme*, which has a very low absorption rate—so even if you eat plenty, your body can use only a small fraction (about 4 percent), and plant-based zinc absorption is also poor. Plus, when inorganic iron is added as a means to "fortify" certain foods, it further blocks zinc absorption! (However, natural forms of animal-based iron do not block zinc.)

Animal foods are the better choice to ensure critical nutrient needs are met. The highly absorbable form of iron, called heme iron, is absorbed at 37 to 40 percent, and it is only found in animal foods. Easily absorbable zinc, too, is found only in animal foods. The animal foods' versions of these nutrients are so well absorbed that even if they are consumed with blockers, they can still be somewhat absorbed.

A HIGH-FAT DIET IS CRITICAL FOR BABIES

When the actual nutritional needs of an infant are reviewed, it is apparent that saturated fat and cholesterol are absolutely *necessary* in a baby's diet! In fact, mom's milk has a caloric make up of 50 to 60 percent fat, over half of which is saturated fat with hefty doses of cholesterol. One of the early enzymes your baby produces is lipase, which enables him to absorb critical fats. Additionally, your mammary glands secrete a substance that ensures your baby best absorbs the cholesterol from your milk. Mother Nature did not make a mistake here, but meant to guarantee with this much saturated fat and cholesterol that your baby's growth and development needs were met. It might interest you to know that your baby's rapidly growing brain is 60 percent fat—being built by fats in his diet.

Experts agree that low-fat, low-cholesterol diets do not provide babies the basis for proper growth. Science supports that babies need most of their calories from fats in the first year, and U.S. governing agencies such as the Food and Drug Administration (FDA) and American Academy of Pediatrics (AAP) agree that babies should not be on any kind of fat-restrictive diet for at least the first 2 years. (In fact, experts in the United Kingdom recommend higher-fat diets for the first 5 years, during which time 80 percent of brain growth occurs.)

The truth about saturated fat and cholesterol. Just as we rave about and crave the benefits of antioxidants, vitamins, minerals, and "good" fats in foods, we should applaud the health benefits of natural cholesterol and saturated fat in foods. Steak, butter, and eggs are rich tasting because they are rich in nutrition. Newer science and newer review of old science has shown that these dietary components have been falsely accused of robbing us of our health. In fact, as saturated fat and cholesterol intake has steadily fallen, diabetes, heart disease, and obesity have been on a steady *incline*.

Cholesterol is a healing agent (like an "internal Band-Aid" or a scab protecting a cut), made daily by your body. Eating cholesterol doesn't clog arteries; rather it serves to help your body by covering damaged areas, such as *inflamed* arteries. Arterial damage isn't from the Band-Aid (cholesterol) but stems from root causes of inflammation (such as sugar and rancid, inflammatory fats) that actually *cause* the damage to arteries. A low-cholesterol diet just forces your body to work harder to make more on its own. In fact, people who don't eat any cholesterol often have the *highest* cholesterol levels, because with none coming in the diet, the body revs up its own production in response. On the contrary, consuming high levels of cholesterol will allow the body to reduce its own production and normalize to only what is needed for good health.

Cholesterol is also:

▸ An antioxidant and fights lipid peroxidation ("brain rusting")

▸ Important for cellular, nervous system, and brain communication

▸ Needed to make hormones and for vitamin D metabolism

▸ Necessary to protect the nervous system and brain

▸ Critical for proper digestive health, intestinal wall integrity, and leaky gut prevention

Fats have also falsely been blamed for poor health; let's discuss a few fat facts to clear up confusion. Four main classes of fats exist: saturated, monounsaturated, polyunsaturated, and trans fats. The three listed first each serve natural health benefits and offer unique fatty acids, required for optimal health. Thus, it is good to include each in your diet, including saturated fats. Trans fats, however, have a man-altered molecular structure that is harmful to health and must be avoided.

Saturated fat is necessary for the following:

▸ Cell structure and integrity of all the cell walls that make up your baby's body
▸ Absorption and use of fat-soluble nutrients (vitamins E and K1, beta-carotene, lycopene, zeaxanthin, lutein, CoQ10, etc.)
▸ Ensuring mineral activators (vitamins A, D3, K2) get assimilated and therefore minerals are absorbed
▸ Proper brain development
▸ Building nervous system communication components
▸ Absorption, conversion, and use of key nutrients
▸ Aiding in important metabolic functions of the body
▸ Uniquely providing short-, medium-, and long-chain fatty acids
▸ Feeding the heart (its preferred fuel is saturated fat)
▸ Supporting health of lung tissue
▸ Ensuring bone strength and health
▸ As a source of antimicrobial and antiviral agents in the digestive tract
▸ *Reducing* your need for as many omega-3s to do important inflammatory work because saturated fats make omega-3s more "efficient"

Contemporary First Foods Challenge Your Baby's Health

Your baby is growing more rapidly in his first year than he will at any other time in his life. His need for nutrients during this time is significant and mustn't be underestimated. Consequently, it is critical that those first baby foods contain all the nutrients your baby needs right now.

According to pediatricians, the media, and maybe even your family and friends, first foods should be rice cereal, yellow then green vegetables, then fruits and other grains, like oatmeal. Yet surprisingly, these common "baby" foods don't contain enough of the specific nutrients that babies at this age absolutely require. Furthermore, they don't provide adequate energy and are rough on babies' still-developing digestive systems.

BABIES ARE FUNCTIONALLY GRAIN INTOLERANT

Your baby's body is not ready to digest grains. Though he does produce lactase to break down milk sugar (lactose), he doesn't yet make other enzymes to digest additional carbohydrates. Closer to one year of age, babies begin making amylase, but a more complete set of carbohydrate enzymes won't be present until approximately 3 years of age. Some carbohydrates (like fiber) can never be digested by humans, since we don't ever produce the right enzymes; thus, we must rely on our friendly intestinal flora ("probiotics") to digest them for us.

Since food intolerance can be defined as not having the proper enzymes to digest a food, babies (prior to toddlerhood) are functionally grain intolerant because they don't effectively make starch-digesting enzymes. As they have not yet built up sufficient beneficial bacterial colonies, babies are also fiber intolerant.

RICE CEREAL ISN'T RIGHT

Rice cereal flakes are a refined grain, which has been stripped of natural nutrients. Such cereal is hardly more than sugar to your baby's body. Iron-fortified cereal offers only a 4 percent absorption rate for iron, and that form of iron makes zinc absorption worse. So while the label might look nutritious, the rice flakes inside aren't, and they don't provide the critical nutrients and calories your baby needs.

In general, whole grains are better than refined. But before you take the "brown rice flakes" off the grocery store shelf or go for oatmeal, here's a news flash on whole grains: In addition to being very hard to digest, they block critical mineral absorption. According to a study in the *Journal of Nutrition*, low levels of zinc are most often found in diets that have a lot of whole grains (wheat, corn, rice, oatmeal) and legumes, like soy. Such foods contain an antinutrient called phytic acid, which blocks not only zinc but also calcium, magnesium, and iron from being absorbed. (Note that grains *can* be part of a healthful diet for older babies. See chapter 6.)

FRUITS AND VEGGIES ALONE WON'T DO

The other common choice for initial feeding is fruits and veggies. While these foods do have antioxidants and other nutrients, they contain significantly less amino acids, vitamins, and critical minerals than do animal-based foods and therefore shouldn't be relied on to provide optimal, protective nutrition for babies. Also, as low-calorie foods, they're a poor choice for the *increasing* caloric demands of growing babies.

Traditional First Foods Offer Super Nutrition

If grains, cereals, fruits, and vegetables don't contain enough of what your baby needs, then what do you feed him? Ideally, your baby's first foods will contain protein, fat, cholesterol, and plenty of absorbable iron and zinc—just like mom's milk! Such nutrients are found all together in only one type of food: animal-source foods that include beef, lamb, organ meat, eggs, poultry, fish, and fresh dairy.

Are you surprised? For some, these recommendations might be eyebrow raising. Yet according to the professional textbook *Nutrition in Pediatrics: Basic Science, Clinical Applications*, "Incorporating animal source foods . . . is often the *only* way to supply . . . [adequate] nutrients through natural foods." [emphasis added] The AAP likewise recommends animal foods as first foods and suggests "pureed meats as good first foods because they contain ample protein, iron and zinc."

Despite the research and AAP recommendations, parents are still most often instructed to feed their babies rice cereal, fruits, and veggies as first foods. Yet animal foods are the perfect first food for babies. (Mom's milk is actually your baby's first animal food.)

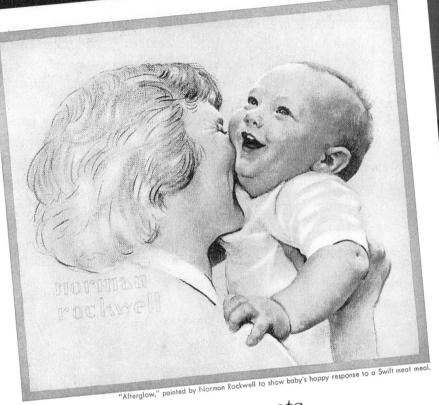

"Afterglow," painted by Norman Rockwell to show baby's happy response to a Swift meat meal.

Swift's new <u>smoother</u> meats are easy to <u>enjoy</u>...easy to <u>digest</u>!

● Held in the haven of your arms, baby's aglow with a warm feeling of well-being after a happy feeding of the new Swift's Meats. And your peace of mind is complete in these precious moments of shared contentment.

How satisfying . . . the wonderful flavors and creamy-smooth texture of Swift's Strained Meats! They feel soft as velvet on baby's delicate tongue and they're just as digestible as milk.

How comforting for you to know these fine 100% meats are just as good *for* your baby as they taste. Abundantly rich in proteins, vitamins and minerals, they help build strong bones and good red blood.

Why don't you let Swift's Meats help provide the foundation for good health for *your* baby? There are 8 varieties to serve— all tempting in flavor and brimful of natural meat nourishment. Remember Swift's Egg Yolks, too—for vitamin A and iron.

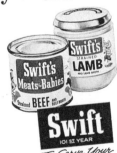

MEATS FOR BABIES
Swift's most precious product

HEALTH BENEFITS OF ANIMAL FOODS
AS FIRST FOODS

Animal foods are higher in age-critical minerals than are grains, fruits, and veggies. Research from the *Journal of Nutrition* confirms, "Animal source foods can provide a variety of micronutrients that are difficult to obtain in adequate quantities from plant source foods alone." Animal foods are so nutrient dense, they require *fewer* calories to provide rich nutrition compared to plant foods. Here are additional characteristics of animal-source foods that make them so important for your baby.

All essential amino acids. Your baby needs eight *essential* amino acids from his diet because he can't make them (neither can adults). These are necessary to build his body, including making heart, lung, and intestinal tissue, other muscles, antibodies, hormones, neurotransmitters, enzymes, bones, ligaments, tendons, cell membranes, and more! All eight are found together in animal foods, but *not* in plant foods.

Unique nutrients not found elsewhere. Animal foods, but not plants, supply taurine, carnitine, CoQ10, vitamin A (retinol), B12, conjugated linoleic acid (CLA), butyric acid, carnosine, long-chain superunsaturated fatty acids (AA, EPA, and DHA), cholesterol, and vitamin D3.

Bioavailable form of nutrients. Animal foods also offer nutrients, like B6, iron, zinc, magnesium, copper, and calcium, in a particularly "body-ready" form that is easily absorbed and used by your baby.

Animal foods provide antioxidants. While fruits and veggies get all the glory for antioxidants, very powerful antioxidants like superoxide dismutase, glutathione, carnosine, CoQ10, and carnitine are made from nutrients in animal foods.

Animal foods allow for lower calories to meet nutrient needs. Contrary to popular belief, animal foods provide more nutrition in *fewer* calories and significantly smaller quantities than plant sources to get the same nutrition. (See chart on opposite page and sidebar on page 50.) Per calorie, animal foods are more nutrient dense.

Animal foods are better digested. The first readily available digestive enzymes your baby makes are those for digesting protein, fat, and cholesterol. Perhaps this is why, historically, traditional first baby foods have always been animal based.

Feed Animal Foods for Strong, Smart, and Social Children

Numerous studies reported in several major American and European medical journals reveal that animal-source foods are integral to adequate growth, musculature, activity levels, and cognitive development in growing children.

Specifically, a study reported in the *Journal of Nutrition*, found that children eating meat had 80 percent greater increase in upper-arm muscle. The meat-eating group also scored higher on intelligence tests, which has been corroborated by several studies to date. According to researchers, the meat eaters were also "more active on the playground, more talkative and playful, and showed more leadership skills."

Comparing Nutrient Richness of Produce to Animal Foods

Nutrient	Apple (100 g)	Carrots (100 g)	Red Meat (100 g)	Beef Liver (100 g)
Calcium	3.0 mg	3.3 mg	11.0 mg	11.0 mg
Phosphorus	6.0 mg	31.0 mg	140.0 mg	476.0 mg
Magnesium	4.8 mg	6.2 mg	15.0 mg	18.0 mg
Potassium	139.0 mg	222.0 mg	370.0 mg	380.0 mg
Iron	0.1 mg	0.6 mg	3.3 mg	8.8 mg
Zinc	0.05 mg	0.3 mg	4.4 mg	4.0 mg
Copper	0.04 mg	0.08 mg	0.18 mg	12.0 mg
Vitamin A	None	None	40 IU	53,400 IU
Vitamin D	None	None	Trace	19 IU
Vitamin E	0.37 mg	0.11 mg	1.7 mg	0.63 mg
Vitamin C	7.0 mg	6.0 mg	None	27.0 mg
Thiamine	0.03 mg	0.05 mg	0.05 mg	0.26 mg
Riboflavin	0.02 mg	0.05 mg	0.20 mg	4.19 mg
Niacin	0.10 mg	0.60 mg	4.0 mg	16.5 mg
Pantothenic acid	0.11 mg	0.19 mg	0.42 mg	8.8 mg
Vitamin B6	0.03 mg	0.10 mg	0.07 mg	0.73 mg
Folic acid	8.0 mcg	24.0 mcg	4.0 mcg	145.0 mcg
Biotin	None	0.42 mcg	2.8 mcg	96.0 mcg
Vitamin B12	None	None	1.84 mcg	111.3 mcg

Reprinted with permission from Chris Kresser's nutrition information blog, http://thehealthyskeptic.org.
Note: 100 grams is just under 1 cup of apple (1 cup = 125 grams), under a cup of carrots (1 cup = 128 grams), and is about 3.5 ounces (1 ounce = 28 grams) of ground beef or liver.

Further research demonstrates that children eating animal foods also grow stronger bones and are taller and even leaner. Milk and meat significantly increase the height of schoolchildren, making them grow faster, and even can correct stunted growth.

VEGETARIANISM ISN'T THE "HEALTHIEST"

All this talk of animal foods . . . but aren't diets based on plant foods the best? The answer is emphatically: No! Grains, greens, beans, and soy-based diets are *not* nutritionally adequate and certainly miss the mark on optimal nourishment for your growing baby.

Plant-based diets have mineral blockers, enzyme inhibitors, protein digestion blockers, poorly absorbed minerals, digestive irritants, are often inflammatory, tend to be high in sugars, and are nearly always lacking and deficient in nutrients critical for healthy growth and development. Diets free of animal foods include low levels of, or less available, nutrients such as the following:

- Vitamin A and D (fat-soluble activators), resulting in poor mineral usage
- Body-ready essential fatty acids (AA, EPA, and DHA, necessary for brain and cognitive development, immune support, and anti-inflammation)
- CoQ10 (necessary for fighting free radicals; aids the cardiovascular system)
- Cholesterol (necessary for brain development and cellular communication)
- Body-ready B6 (necessary for several conversions of happiness neurotransmitters and aids in detoxification pathways; also helps B12 and folic acid convert harmful homocysteine—a risk factor in cardiovascular disease)
- B12 (soy further increases the need for B12)
- Body-ready zinc and iron
- Amino acids (carnitine, taurine, carnosine, necessary for fighting free radicals, inflammation, and are very helpful for cardiovascular health, aid in fat metabolism and cellular energy production, and protect the eyes and the brain)

Several researchers have found that animal foods are so important in ensuring proper growth and height, strength, and intelligence, they contest it is unhealthy *not* to include animal foods in children's diets. And vegan diets fare even worse: After extensive research on the criticality of animal foods on children's health, Lindsay Allen, Ph.D., professor in the program in international nutrition at the University of California, Davis, states, "There's absolutely no question that it's unethical for parents to bring up their children as strict vegans." (For the vegetarian nursing mother, we strongly recommend beginning your baby on solid foods no later than 6 months.)

We respect the beliefs of many vegetarians and are equally appalled by the cruel and unjust treatment of factory-farmed animals. Yet we still strongly recommend parents provide the best-quality *animal foods* available for feeding their babies at this critical young age. By procuring animal foods from pastured farms, you will both be supporting animal husbandry that is humane, healthiest, and happiest for the animals *and* be providing foods with superior nutritional content.

CHOOSE PASTURED ANIMAL FOODS

We *strongly* advocate procuring animal foods for your baby from pastured sources, where the animals are not confined, but free to roam, follow their instincts, self-select their diet from nature, and employ their natural immune system with fresh air and sunshine.

Both the quality of life and the nutrient profile of such animals are vastly superior to those that come from the factory-farming model.

Benefits of pasture-based animal foods. Pasture-based and "grass-fed" refer to the methods of feeding that allow animals to eat their natural diets based on their nutritional instincts. Cows on pasture eat grass and clover; pigs eat bark, foliage, and small animals; chickens eat bugs, worms, and weeds. Animals on pasture:

▸ Can vary their natural diet as they need to meet their needs
▸ Are exposed to fresh air and sunlight—activating vitamin D synthesis and supporting their natural immune system (they're healthier)
▸ Experience calmer, more natural lives
▸ Have the best fats and fatty-acid ratios (omega-3 to omega-6)
▸ Provide significantly more nutrients as food

Super Nutrition Food Categorizations for 6 to 8 Months

Super POWER	PURE
Grated frozen liver	Organic avocado
Soft-boiled egg yolks (warm but runny) from organic, free-range, pastured hens	Organic soup stock–braised vegetables
Marrow, from grass-fed organic bones	Organic peeled, stewed, puréed fruits with fat
Souper Stock (page 56), from grass-fed organic animals	Organic banana
High-quality, high-vitamin cod liver oil, preferably fermented	Souper Stock (page 56) from organic animals
	Soft-boiled organic egg yolks, omega-3 fortified
	Grass-fed, organic meats

OKAY	CRAP
Organic baby food jars (stage 1 to 2)	Teething biscuits
Nonorganic avocado	Rice flakes
Nonorganic banana	Brown rice flakes
Nonorganic vegetables (washed, prepared in stock)	Oatmeal or other grains
Souper Stock (page 56) from nonorganic animals	Soy anything
	Nonorganic baby food
	Juice (organic and nonorganic)

Make It a Liver and Swiss; Hold the Supersized Brown Rice and Broccoli

To meet the RDA for calcium (1,000 mg) you can eat 50 cups (9.8 kg) of brown rice (10,800 calories), 100 ounces (2.8 kg) of tofu (1,500 calories), 3 cups (435 g) of almonds (2,225 calories), or just under 4 ounces (112 g) of Swiss cheese (482 calories).

The RDA for iron (8 mg for men, higher for women) can be met by 20 cups (600 g) of spinach (only 140 calories, but who can eat 20 cups of spinach?), 25 cups (1.8 kg) of broccoli (775 calories), 5 cups (775 g) of edamame (945 calories), or 5 ounces (140 g) of liver (240 calories).

Real Foods Offer Super Nutrition

Real foods, as described in chapter 1, are those as nature intended them. They are in whole form, grown naturally, preferably local and seasonal, vine ripened, raw and not pasteurized, pastured and not factory farmed, and without additional chemicals. Such foods maintain some of their enzyme content, making them more digestible—which is of critical importance at this age. Hard-to-digest foods lead to a host of health problems that could easily be avoided by making smart early-foods choices. With the recipes that follow, we'll take you far from fake flakes to real, nourishing, digestible foods for your baby.

PRACTICAL FEEDING TIPS AT THIS AGE

Most medical and scientific experts recommend feeding babies only mom's milk or formula until age 6 months. Further, the World Health Organization and the AAP state not to introduce *any* solids before 4 months of age.

Before 6 months your baby:

- Doesn't make enzymes needed to digest first foods
- Has underdeveloped kidneys, not yet ready to handle waste from solids
- Is lacking sufficient beneficial bacteria required for digestion
- Has an "open" gut, which means if solid foods are introduced too soon, they could increase the risk of food allergies (see page 39)

For these reasons, it is best to wait until at least 6 months of age *and* until your baby shows all the signs that he's ready for solids. Does your baby meet the following criteria?

- Sits unassisted or with minimal support
- When something comes toward his mouth or face, he opens his mouth
- Can indicate disinterest in further feeding by turning his head away
- Closes lips around a spoon when introduced to mouth
- Seems interested when others are eating, watching food travel from plate to mouth

It starts young and never goes ~

this natural, healthful craving for Campbell's Tomato Soup!

The child's quick, alert taste responds instantly to the gay flavor of Campbell's Tomato Soup. Nature paints the tomato a flaming scarlet to catch the eye and tempt the taste to one of her most precious foods. The instinctive eagerness of children for a flavor that sparkles and tingles with fresh, vivacious goodness is revealed by their universal fondness for Campbell's Tomato Soup. You may indulge them with it freely.

For Campbell's Tomato Soup is a product so wholesome, so uniform, so scientifically protected in every step of its making that the most exacting mothers have implicit faith in its quality and safety. When you want it extra-nourishing for the children, why not mix it with milk instead of water, according to the easy directions on the label? Get a supply of Campbell's Tomato Soup today.

LOOK FOR THE RED-AND-WHITE LABEL

21 kinds to choose from . . .

Asparagus
Bean
Beef
Bouillon
Celery
Chicken
Chicken-Gumbo
Clam Chowder
Consommé
Julienne
Mock Turtle
Mulligatawny
Mutton
Ox Tail
Pea
Pepper Pot
Printanier
Tomato
Tomato-Okra
Vegetable
Vegetable-Beef
Vermicelli-Tomato

11 cents a can

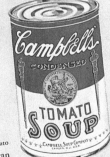

Campbell's CONDENSED TOMATO SOUP

CAMPBELL SOUP COMPANY, CAMDEN, N.J., U.S.A.

Oh boy, just see
My manly muscle!
Eat Campbell's Soup
For vim and hustle!

MEAL-PLANNING IS EASIER WITH DAILY CHOICES FROM CAMPBELL'S 21 SOUPS

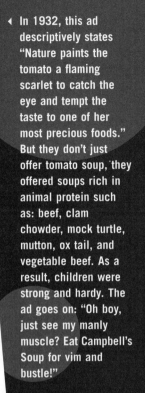

◀ In 1932, this ad descriptively states "Nature paints the tomato a flaming scarlet to catch the eye and tempt the taste to one of her most precious foods." But they don't just offer tomato soup, they offered soups rich in animal protein such as: beef, clam chowder, mock turtle, mutton, ox tail, and vegetable beef. As a result, children were strong and hardy. The ad goes on: "Oh boy, just see my manly muscle? Eat Campbell's Soup for vim and bustle!"

Very-first meals. First meals can simply be offered between regular feeding times or instead offered after a shortened nursing session or a smaller bottle. When you first introduce solids, you don't want your baby to be starving and therefore frustrated, nor too full to be interested.

Consistency and texture. "Solid" foods shouldn't be solid. Use mom's milk, homemade or enriched formula (chapter 8), or Souper Stock (page 56) to thin foods to the right consistency for your child. The consistency should graduate in thickness and texture as your baby seems ready.

Water? Extra water to drink isn't necessary during 6 to 8 months of age, as your baby should get enough fluid from mom's milk or formula. If it is hot and everyone else is thirsty, then an ounce or two (28 to 60 ml) of water can be offered from a cup or bottle. Your baby should be nursing about six to eight times a day or be drinking 28 to 32 ounces (805 to 950 ml) a day of homemade or enriched formula to ensure adequate hydration.

What's enough? Let your baby be the guide in what he wants to eat and how much is enough. When he turns away or is no longer interested, the meal is over.

Farm Cooperatives and Consumer-Supported Agriculture (CSA)

While health food stores can provide grass-fed animal foods, often a better place to get your animal foods is from a local, trusted, pasture-based farm.

Farm co-ops are available in most areas, where simply emailing in a weekly or monthly order allows you to meet at the drop spot, cut a check, and take home your nutritious, fresh food. You can find local, pastured, organic animal foods, as well as trusted raw dairy farmers, near you by contacting your local chapter of the Weston A. Price Foundation (www.westonaprice.org) or by searching "buy fresh buy local" on the Internet.

For produce, we recommend joining a CSA (visit www.localharvest.org to find one near you). Getting fresh, local, seasonal, and organic produce from a CSA saves money, supports your local economy, increases variety, and provides nutritional benefits. Due to very short transportation routes, fruits and vegetables are vine ripened, enabling them to get a last infusion of nutrition from the soil (unlike foods from your grocery store, which ripen on the shelf). Additionally, produce is often harvested the same day that it is delivered, substantially increasing the enzyme content of the food.

Slow introduction. Introduce new foods every 3 to 4 days so that you can observe any possible allergic reactions. Preferably, give new foods earlier in the day (rather than before bedtime).

Pattern, not schedule. Establish a repeatable pattern, such as nursing upon waking, midmorning meal, nursing before afternoon nap, dinner with the family, and nursing before bed. Following a *pattern*, as opposed to randomly feeding or being on a strict, clock-based schedule, will allow you to offer a critical sense of meal reliability for your baby, while still allowing some flexibility in your day.

Recipes for Real Foods Offering Optimal Nourishment

For the initial foods that your baby will digest all by himself, we present "very-first foods" that will adequately aid his digestion, provide him with optimal nutrition, and will not cause him intestinal distress. After a few weeks of these foods, you can introduce additional "first foods."

FEEDING VERY-FIRST FOODS AT 6 MONTHS

As you begin your baby on food, continue nursing or feeding homemade or enriched formula (see chapter 8). Provide regular feedings, as before, with a shortened session at the new "meal" times. In the first few weeks of feeding, you can introduce soft-boiled egg yolk, liver, Souper Stock (page 56), and some minimal braised meat with the stock. For a complete list of acceptable foods at this age, see the Food Introduction Timeline on page 222.

Pattern	First 2 Weeks of Meals
Early AM	Milk / homemade formula (upon waking)
Mid-Morning	Very-first foods
Mid-Day	Milk / homemade formula
Afternoon	Milk / homemade formula (before nap)
Evening	Milk / homemade formula
Nighttime	Milk / homemade formula (before bed)

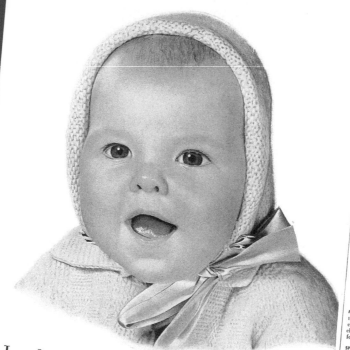

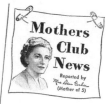

Look who's started loving liver!

What about your baby? Does he smack his lips when you offer that important Vitamin A food—liver? Until *you* see and taste Gerber's Liver, you can't possibly know it hasn't even a trace of the usual liver bitterness. Ummm! *This* good-for-Baby meat really tastes good.

And oh, the luscious Beef and Veal Gerber's bring your young hopeful. You'll see, every spoonful has true meat flavor—and color. Yes, years of preparing *only* baby foods, have taught us that even tiny infants prefer foods that look, taste and "feel" good on the tongue.

The sooner the better! The very week your doctor says, "Start your baby on protein-rich meats"—get Gerber's Meats. They're oh-so-carefully prepared for your infant or toddler. Every spoonful is selected Armour Beef, Veal or Liver. So look for the famous Gerber Baby on wonderful meats—and everything from Starting Cereals through Strained and Junior Foods.

ARMOUR

Gerber's
BABY FOODS
Fremont, Mich.

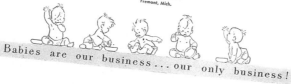

Babies are our business...our only business!

Soft-Boiled Egg Yolk

Mom's milk and eggs yolks provide the "perfect protein" for babies, containing an ideal suite of vitamins, minerals, and amino acids, along with the enzymes to help break them down. Known as "brain food" the world over, egg yolks are the ideal first food.

Why serve soft-boiled? Animal foods are very rich in heat-sensitive enzymes, but overcooking destroys them, reducing their digestibility and making the food more allergenic. Also, cooking the yolk until firm makes it dry and chalky, and your baby won't swallow it as easily as a warm, runny yolk.

1 high-quality egg (see sidebar on next page)
Pinch (less than ¹/₈ teaspoon) Celtic sea salt

In a small saucepan, boil water. Using a spoon, slip in the egg. Lower the heat to just below its highest setting, but continuing to boil the water, and cook the egg for 3¹/₂ to 4 minutes.

Remove the egg from water with a spoon and drop in a bowl to crack it (it will be very hot). When the egg is open, peel away some white, which is semihard. The yolk should slip out in a malleable ball. Scoop up the yolk with a spoon and put into a different small bowl, leaving all the white behind.

The yolk should be warm and soft, not firm or "dry." Add sea salt to supply additional trace minerals and improve taste (see discussion of salt in chapter 6). Spoon-feed it to your baby.

Yield: 1 egg yolk

Liver

Liver is the best source of almost all known nutrients—a veritable powerhouse of nutrition. In addition to the zinc and iron your baby needs in first foods, liver is the best source of copper. It also has brain-building choline, anti-inflammatory omega-3s (particularly if from grass-fed sources), serotonin-making tryptophan, and is rich in antioxidants. Best of all, babies love it!

2 teaspoons raw liver (grated if frozen, or finely minced if refrigerated)
1 tablespoon (14 g) ghee, coconut oil, or (13 g) lard
2 tablespoons (28 ml) Souper Stock (page 56)

Sauté the liver in fat over low heat for 1 to 2 minutes—liver should be a pinkish brown when done. Off heat, mash and thin with the stock to desired consistency.

Optional: Mix the liver into your baby's daily egg yolk, mom's milk (or with other foods as you add them) for a fortifying, nutritionally superior meal. For more early baby-feeding information, including using grated liver for your baby, visit www.westonaprice.org and enter "Nourishing a Growing Baby" in the search engine.

Yield: 1 serving

Notes
- Very little liver is needed for a super nutrition boost—start with just ¹/₂ to 1 teaspoon.
- Due to the high quantity of vitamin A found in liver, limit your baby to 1 chicken liver or 1 ounce (28 g) of beef/calf liver every other day; or 10 grams of liver (¹/₃ to ¹/₂ ounce) per day on average, particularly if you're providing cod liver oil.

Does the Kind of Egg Matter?

Eggs from pastured chickens on a local farm will have as much inflammation-fighting omega-3s as wild-caught salmon, as well as more vitamin A, more beta-carotene, and more brain-building long-chain fatty acids that support mental development and sharp vision.

Choosing the highest-quality, organic, free-range, +omega-3 eggs, freshest from a farm co-op, will substantially decrease the already-low (1 in 30,000 eggs) chances of salmonella contamination (most outbreaks of salmonella aren't related to eggs at all) and provide 30 to 40 percent higher DHA. DHA is a critical omega-3 essential fatty acid, well recognized for its benefits in cognitive development and functioning.

- If you can't get clean liver, another option is to add powdered, dessicated liver to your baby's meals or mix with mom's milk or formula. Find grass-fed, dessicated liver capsules at www.radiantlifecatalog.com. Six capsules is equivalent to 1 ounce (28 g) of liver.
- Contrary to commonly held beliefs, healthy liver does not store toxins but rather processes and converts them so they can be excreted. A fatty liver in sick animals, however, *will* contain toxins, since toxins are stored in fatty tissue, wheras healthy livers are lean.

Souper Stock

Real soup, made from bones, is excellent for the digestive system because it contains gelatin, which is uniquely able to stimulate and support digestion, making whatever you eat with it easier to digest. The minerals obtained from soup stock made with bones are extremely nutritious and in highly absorbable form, resulting in an electrolyte (mineral) solution far superior to Pedialyte or Gatorade.

1 to 2 pounds (455 to 910 g) marrow bones, knuckle bones, oxtail, or soup bones from organic, grass-fed animals (beef, lamb, or poultry)

2 tablespoons (28 ml) vinegar (white distilled, raw apple cider, or brown rice)

In a slow cooker, soak the bones for 1 hour in the vinegar, adding enough water to cover. This helps to leach minerals from the bones.

Add enough water to fill the pot and simmer on low for 12 to 72 hours (the longer the bones simmer, the more minerals and gelatin will be present in your stock).

Let cool. Add a pinch (less than 1/8 teaspoon) of Celtic sea salt into a serving for flavor and to provide trace minerals (see discussion of salt in chapter 4).

Serve warm to your baby.

Allow to cool in the refrigerator and then skim off the fat that rises and firms as a top layer. (This fat can be saved and later used to sauté liver.)

Yield: 3 quarts (2.8 L)

Note

- The acidity in the water helps to pull minerals from the bones, but too much vinegar will alter the taste of the broth; typically 1 tablespoon (15 ml) to 1/2 cup (120 ml) of vinegar is used, depending on the amount of water.

Storage:

- Pour through a mesh strainer into either mason jars or ice-cube trays as an option for freezing individual serving sizes.
- For use within a week or two, place in refrigerator; otherwise, freeze. If frozen and defrosted, use within 3 to 4 days.
- When refrigerated, Souper Stock should be gelatinous (jiggly like Jell-O).

Mom to Mom / Make Souper Stock every other weekend and use frozen in between. If you run out, you can use Bernard Jensen's unbleached gelatin found at www.radiantlifecatalog.com sprinkled into filtered water to eat with small amounts of puréed meat. Digestion will still be aided, though the important minerals will be absent.

Braised Lamb and Souper Stock

As lamb is not as mass-produced as beef, it tends to be from grass-fed sources. Red meat like lamb is a great source of heme iron (the absorbable kind) and other minerals.

3/4 pound (340 g) fresh lamb meat (shoulder chops or lamb steaks are ideal)

1 recipe Souper Stock (page 56), in progress

Add the lamb meat to your slow cooker with the simmering stock.

After simmering for 2 to 4 hours, spoon out a few teaspoons of meat and purée. Thin with the stock, using a hand blender or regular blender. (Have caution when blending hot liquids.)

Yield: Dinner for two adults and baby, or 6 to 8 baby servings

As this 1934 ad pronounces, vitamin D—from high-quality cod liver oil—will help children "develop a well-proportioned framework" including "well-shaped heads, fine, full chests, strong backs, and straight legs." This is true, as minerals that build teeth and skeletal "framework" require vitamin D to activate them. Also, the ad correctly says: Cod liver oil provides "not only vitamin D, but the resistance-building, growth-promoting factor—vitamin A." These claims still hold true today, though this nutritional wisdom has been lost over the last few generations—but parents today should also want their babies to be "vitamin protected." Children would be much better off if parents renewed their grandmother's practice of giving a daily dose of cod liver oil!

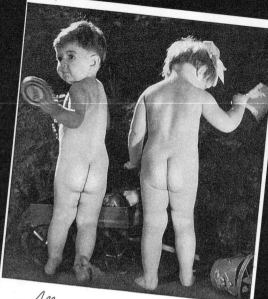

All summer the sun helps them build strong backs, full chests, straight legs..... But now especially they need BOTTLED SUNSHINE!

Outdoors the sun shining on their bare little bodies helps them develop a well-proportioned framework. The important factor produced by sunshine – Vitamin D – also helps them build sound, even, well-spaced teeth.

This is why physicians insist that babies be given sun baths outdoors *every day* all summer.

But now that seasonal factors such as clouds, smoke, fog, clothing and ordinary window glass interfere, mothers are urged to give them an *inner* sun bath daily! With *Bottled Sunshine* – good cod-liver oil!

Good cod-liver oil supplies an abundance of bone-and-tooth building Vitamin D! Babies who get it regularly every day are helped to develop well-shaped heads, fine, full chests, strong backs, and straight legs....

In addition, good cod-liver oil keeps up their resistance and helps them to grow. It provides, not only Vitamin D, but the resistance-building, growth-promoting factor – *Vitamin A.*

Not all cod-liver oils, though, are equally rich in Vitamins A and D. Some are so much more effective than others!

This is why hundreds of mothers always ask for the kind they know is vitamin-protected – Squibb's Cod-Liver Oil!

How protecting vitamin content as Squibb does means a saving to mothers.... Vitamin protection in cod-liver oil amounts to just this. Each teaspoonful contains more Vitamins A and D than inferior kinds! With a small dose, the baby gets greater help. One bottle goes much further. Always insist on the *best* cod-liver oil. It's actually the least expensive! For your baby – *every day* – Squibb's.

Is there a tiny baby in the family?.... Try Squibb's "10 D" Oil! Richer than regular cod-liver oil in bone-and-tooth building Vitamin D, it is especially suited to the needs of rapidly growing young babies. When you ask for it, give the full name – *Squibb's Cod-Liver Oil with Viosterol-10 D.*

Older children like the Mint Flavored and it helps keep them well!.... They will have greater resistance this winter if you give it to them regularly every day. They like its pleasant taste.

Free..Booklet for mothers! 'Why Every Baby Needs Bottled Sunshine.' Write E. R. Squibb & Sons, 745 Fifth Ave., New York.

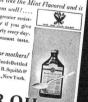

SQUIBB'S COD·LIVER OIL

VITAMIN-TESTED AND VITAMIN-PROTECTED.... Produced, tested, and *guaranteed by E. R. Squibb & Sons, manufacturing chemists to the medical profession since 1858*

Bottled Sunshine

Cod Liver Oil

In 2011, the AAP journal, Pediatrics, *reported on the importance of DHA (an essential omega-3 fatty acid as found in Cod Liver Oil) for infants and its critical role in reducing infant morbidity (deaths)! Cod liver oil (CLO) not only provides DHA, but also has a super combination of the special fat-soluble vitamins A and D3 (which are necessary for utilizing minerals), as well as inflammation-fighting fatty acids. It helps the nervous system function, supports cellular communication, and assists in the colonization of probiotics in the gut. Fermented CLO additionally provides vitamin K2, necessary for helping vitamins A and D3 in the absorption and utilization of minerals. Since it has twice the vitamin A and D3 of regular cod liver oil, only half the amount is needed. If you're not using fermented CLO, we recommend butter oil in conjunction with a high-vitamin CLO. For brands, see the Weston A. Price Foundation shopping guide (see Resources, page 218).*

Dosing:

¹/₂ to 1 teaspoon high-quality cod liver oil, or ¹/₄ to ¹/₂ teaspoon fermented cod liver oil (¹/₂ teaspoon = 2.5 milliliters)

Administration: To avoid your baby choking on the oil, it is of the utmost importance that you either mix it in pumped breast milk or formula or give gently by spoon. *Never* squirt oil into your baby's mouth since oil aspiration is very dangerous. Unless mixed in breast milk or formula, don't give CLO before sleep; never give oil to a child who is screaming or fighting; and avoid giving oil to a baby who frequently spits up. Keep babies upright for 15 to 30 minutes after administration.

Notes

- Give CLO particularly on days your baby is not consuming liver or fish roe.
- If you are breast-feeding and taking CLO yourself, your baby will not need supplemental CLO. However, if your baby already has a 3C condition, such as eczema, then it is recommended.
- If you are making homemade formula (see chapter 8), the correct amount of CLO is already within the formula.

FEEDING FIRST FOODS AT 6¹/₂ MONTHS

In the second few weeks of feeding, you can introduce avocado, banana, and poultry-based Souper Stock. Additionally, continue the already-introduced foods from the previous section, possibly adding some small amounts of additional braised meat with the Souper Stock.

Pattern	Second half of 6th month
Early AM	Milk / homemade formula
Mid-Morning	New choice
Mid-Day	Milk / homemade formula
Afternoon	Milk / homemade formula (before nap)
Evening	Already-introduced food
Nighttime	Milk / homemade formula (before bed)

Chicken Soup

Chicken soup is an age-old health food—but hold the noodles. By regularly serving bone-based stocks and soups, you'll be providing necessary minerals in usable form and gelatin that will serve to protect and soothe a digestive tract that is now busy handling new foods!

1 to 2 pounds (455 to 910 g) high-quality whole chicken, including the neck (preferably pasture raised from a local organic farm, otherwise organic, or at least all natural)

1 teaspoon Celtic sea salt

1 to 2 tablespoons (15 to 28 ml) vinegar (raw apple cider vinegar, brown rice vinegar, or white distilled vinegar)

Chicken feet to increase gelatin, optional

Remove the liver and use separately. Gizzards can be added to the stock as it simmers.

Put ingredients in pot and add water to fill. Simmer in your slow cooker or on the stovetop in a stock pot for 6 to 24 hours (longer is better for higher mineral and gelatin content of the stock). Remove the chicken meat from the pot after about two hours (this is so the meat wil not dry out), but allow the bones to continue to simmer. Remove the skin and any bones and strain.

Serve the warm stock to your baby.

Cool the remaining soup in the refrigerator, having strained it into glass storage containers; later remove the firmed-fat top layer. Store in the refrigerator or in individual servings in ice cube trays in the freezer for future use.

Optional: If making chicken soup for your family, add vegetables (such as carrots, onion, parsnips, and celery), but don't yet serve them to your baby.

Yield: Dinner for a family of 4 or 5, or 10 to 12 baby servings

Note

- Remove the majority of the chicken meat after 2 hours of cooking to retain moistness.

Mashed Banana

Bananas' high enzyme content (namely, amylase) means that they can digest themselves and thus, there's less work for your baby's digestive system to do. Choose organic bananas, as sprayed fungicides can reach the fruit inside the porous peel. Also select brown-spotted bananas—they taste the sweetest and are the easiest to digest.

Mash 1/4 peeled banana with a fork and thin with mom's milk or homemade formula (see chapter 8), if necessary.

Mashed Avocado

Avocados are a fabulous source of monounsaturated fats and contain the enzyme lipase, which predigests the avocado's fat as it ripens—great for your baby's developing digestive system. Choose a soft (neither supersquishy nor hard) Haas avocado with dark brown skin.

Slice the avocado in half all the way around; then, holding each half in your hands, twist the halves apart. Cut away any brown spots.

Store the part that "held on" to the pit—it will keep better with the pit in. Cut the remaining half in another half and peel it. Store the other quarter.

Place a peeled quarter (or less) in a bowl and mash with a fork. Add mom's milk or homemade formula (see chapter 8) to thin, if necessary.

FEEDING FIRST FOODS AT AROUND 7 MONTHS

After about 4 weeks of feeding (around 7 months old), tropical fruits, braised root vegetables in stock, and baked vegetables with healthy fats can be added to the menu. For superdigestive nutrition, sweet potatoes and taro can be lacto-fermented (see page 64). Continue to serve foods that have already been introduced.

Pattern	Second half of 6th month
Early AM	Milk / homemade formula
Mid-Morning	New foods (every 3 to 4 days) + already-introduced food
Mid-Day	Milk / homemade formula
Afternoon	Milk / homemade formula (before nap)
Evening	Already-introduced food
Nighttime	Milk / homemade formula (before bed)

Phyto Party Veggies in Souper Stock

Veggies should be well cooked, soft, and mushy before serving. Cooking in soup is a great way to accomplish this. Ideally, veggies should be consumed with fat or Souper Stock (page 56) since much of their antioxidant nutrition is fat soluble and thus less useful without fat. In addition to soaking up minerals, the veggies will become more digestible. Choose carrots, parsnips, or rutabagas. Cook the vegetables in Souper Stock. Mash with a fork and thin with Souper Stock, mom's milk, or homemade formula (see chapter 8).

Tropical Treasures

Typically, fruits and vegetables have lower amounts of enzymes than do rare or raw animal foods (like steak, liver, or soft-boiled eggs). Tropical fruits are the exception in that for a low-calorie food, they are high in enzymes. As babies don't have many carbohydrate-digesting enzymes yet, these foods are great for early feeding since they digest themselves as they ripen. (Avoid cooking tropical fruits, as heat will destroy these enzymes.) Wash all nonorganic fruits and vegetables with a fruit/vegetable wash containing grapefruit seed extract before cutting. Select cantaloupe, mango, or papaya. Peel, cube, and mash with a fork or use an immersion or regular blender. Strain through a mesh strainer for proper consistency for your baby, if necessary.

Sunny Yellow and Orange Baked Vegetables

Some vegetables, like squash and sweet potatoes, are best prepared by baking. They are high in beta-carotene and easy to digest. To ensure the absorption of their fat-soluble nutrients and antioxidants, they should be consumed with additional fats (marrow or ghee are ideal; butter, coconut oil, or red palm oil are also good options).

Stupendous Sauerkraut

Fermented cabbage is extremely nutrient rich, a half cup (71 g) offering 30 percent of the daily value of vitamin C in just six calories. Additional lactic acid, enzymes, and probiotics make this food a perfect digestive aid. Sauerkraut and sauerkraut juice are remarkable at stimulating adequate stomach acidity, which makes them protective against food allergies. A meal of More Magnificent Meats and Souper Stock (page 88) and sauerkraut is extremely nutritious and kind to the digestive system.

4 cups (360 g) finely chopped or grated loosely packed cabbage

2 tablespoons (28 ml) whey (see Homemade Whey, page 64)

2 teaspoons Celtic sea salt

Mix the ingredients and then tamp down in a quart-size mason jar.

Fill with water (about 1 cup [235 ml]), leaving at least 1 inch (2.5 cm) to top of the jar.

Seal and allow to remain at room temperature for 3 days; then move to refrigerator storage.

Notes

- Alternatively, buy unpasteurized sauerkraut, such as Bubbies brand, at the health food store.
- Instead of whey, you can use culture starter from www.bodyecology.com.
- You can spoon ¼ teaspoon of the sauerkraut juice to your baby before cooked meals, particularly when there is a history of 3C conditions in your family.

- If you're nursing, eating sauerkraut with your meals will help improve your digestion, resulting in less heartburn, more nourishment, and fewer immune responses to foods for both you and your baby.
- You can feed finely cut-up bites of sauerkraut to your baby at 10 to 12 months.

Radiant Roots— Lacto-Fermented Style

Sweet potatoes and taro are great options for introducing lacto-fermented foods (refer to "What in the World Is Lacto-Fermentation?" page 64) into your baby's diet because they are soft and starchy. Lacto-fermented foods aid digestion, provide enzymes, and offer increased nutrients, in addition to being a natural source of probiotics.

Fermented or cultured foods often need a "starter" or catalyst for the fermentation process. Lacto-fermentation typically uses whey as the starter.

1 pound (455 g) taro or sweet potato

½ tablespoon Celtic sea salt

2 tablespoons (28 ml) whey (see Homemade Whey, page 64)

Preheat the oven to 325°F (170°C, gas mark 3).

Pierce the taro or sweet potato with a fork and bake for 1½ hours (or until soft). When cooled off, peel. Add in the whey and mash the mixture.

What in the World is Lacto-Fermentation?

Sometimes called pickling, lacto-fermentation does many nutritionally beneficial things all at once. It allows good bacteria to munch on the natural sugars in foods, causing fermentation to happen. This amazing process neutralizes antinutrients, increases enzymes, greatly increases nutrient content, produces even more good bacteria, and literally predigests food. For centuries, foods were preserved via fermentation.

Lactobacillus, the bacteria that causes pickling, is the most pervasive and ubiquitous good bacteria we know of. It is in the air we breathe, the surfaces we touch, and the foods we eat. It is a common probiotic supplement—you'll see several strains that begin with L. (such as L. acidophilus). The L. stands for *lactobacillus*.

Second to pickles, sauerkraut is probably the best known lacto-fermented food. Cabbage, water, and salt, along with the lactobacteria, can "create" sauerkraut through the lacto-fermentation process.

Place the mashed tuber in a glass bowl and cover. Leave for 24 hours on a counter and then move to a mason jar or glass container and store in the refrigerator.

Thin to appropriate consistency with mom's milk or homemade formula (see chapter 8) and then mix with warm marrow, ghee, butter, or coconut oil.

Yield: 4 to 6 baby servings

Note

- Lacto-fermented root vegetables will last at least 1 to 2 weeks in the refrigerator (though if it smells or tastes "bad" it probably is and should be thrown out).

Homemade Whey

Generally, the best lacto-fermentation "starter" is whey from grass-fed, raw (unpasteurized) cow's milk or yogurt. Otherwise, you can sometimes buy whey directly from a pasture-based farm cooperative. In most cases, if raw milk products are not available, whey can be made from organic whole-milk yogurt in a process similar to what follows (see Homemade Whey from Store-Bought Dairy, page 207).

1 container raw milk or raw yogurt

Mom's-milk whey is actually the best option for making lacto-fermented foods for your baby. If you express your milk (even just 3 ounces [90 ml]) and allow it to sit at room temperature (or optionally in the refrigerator) for approximately 1 to 2 days in a clean, sealed container, the milk will separate into a cream layer and yellow liquid beneath (whey). Cool in the refrigerator so the cream "firms up" and remove the cream layer (which can be mixed with fruits as a custom "dessert" for your baby). You can then use your own whey to lacto-ferment

vegetables for your baby. It's just another way for her to get the natural goodness of your milk! Homemade whey can last 2 to 3 months in the refrigerator.

Not much is needed, just a few teaspoons of whey to lacto-ferment the small servings of root vegetables. For example, if you have only 2 teaspoons of your whey, just use $^1/_2$ to $^3/_4$ cup ($^1/_3$ pound or 152 g) of cooked root. (You can use your milk in other recipes, as you feel comfortable, as it is definitely great for your baby!)

Allow the sealed container of milk or yogurt to sit out at room temperature for a few days. It will separate into whey (the yellow liquid you often see on top of yogurt) and milk solids (curds).

Pour the "clabbered" (separated) dairy through several layers of cheesecloth (or a coffee filter) lining a mesh strainer. The yellow whey will filter through, and the curds will be captured in the cheesecloth. This straining often takes 16 to 24 hours.

Whey lasts 6 months in the refrigerator, sealed in a clean container.

Notes

If raw milk or yogurt is unavailable and your family has a history of 3C conditions, it is wise to avoid *pasteurized* dairy until your baby's first birthday. In such cases, the following starters can be used:

- Additional high-quality Celtic sea salt (1 tablespoon or 15 g)
- Culture starter (see Resources, page 218)
- A novel concept—Mommy Whey! (see sidebar)

Allaying common fears. When *raw* dairy (human, cow, or goat) "sits out" at room temperature, wonderful and healthy things happen. The probiotics and enzymes naturally occurring in this nutritious dairy set to work. They pre-digest the sugars in the milk, they multiply (making the cultured dairy or lacto-fermented end-product more rich in enzymes and probiotics), and they increase the overall antioxidant and nutrient content. Lactic acid, which helps digestion, is also produced. Different than pasteurized dairy, which sours if left out of the refrigerator for too long, raw dairy's nutrition is enhanced by a day or two at room temperature. (And don't worry about making whey during the warmer months—hotter temps actually speed up the process.) We do caution, however, that when preparing whey, ensure that your hands, containers, surfaces, and even your breasts are clean so as to avoid pathogenic bacterial contamination.

Miraculous Marrow

Bone marrow is a forgotten dietary treasure, though it has long-been a traditional food for babies (and is one of the easier baby foods to "make"!). It offers much in the way of Super Nutrition as a great source of nutrient-dense fats, which are digested by lipase obtained from mom's milk. Nursing before (or after) a marrow meal makes sense because suckling stimulates lipase production in your baby.

1 pound (455 g) 1- to 2-inch-thick (2.5 to 5 cm) grass-fed, organic beef marrow bones

Preheat the oven to 425°F (220°C, gas mark 7).

Place the bones on a baking sheet and cook for 15 to 20 minutes. The marrow should be moist and shiny.

Hold the bones with an oven mitt and scrape out the marrow with a spoon or fork (or their handles), taking care not to scrape off any bony material. Marrow should be mashable. If it is dry and flaky, finish scraping the marrow out, put it in an oven-safe small bowl, and bake at 400°F (200°C, gas mark 6) for a few more minutes.

Transfer to a cool bowl.

Mash with a fork and feed tiny bits to your baby or thin it with Souper Stock, mom's milk, or homemade formula (see chapter 8). Or use it like butter—as a spread, with vegetables or fruits, and in soups or with meats; it is excellent to mix with soup-based, steamed, or baked vegetables.

Yield: 4 to 5 servings

Notes

- You can also cook marrow bones in soup, getting two meals out of one—rich mineral soup stock as well as the marrow.
- Bone marrow and bone-based stock have a unique smell that may not be familiar if this is a new culinary adventure for you. Even if the smell is unpleasant, marrow and broth should taste delicious (particularly with adequate salt). If either taste spoiled, it might be best to discard and try again.

> **Mom to Mom /** Avoid nitrates and nitrites. Found in most processed meat products, nitrates and nitrites convert to potent carcinogens called nitrosamines. Read ingredients and avoid food with "sodium nitrate." Since toxic nitrosamines can form in certain cooked foods during storage, don't store and reheat dishes of nonorganic carrots, beets, turnips, and spinach. Fortunately, lacto-fermented foods and Souper Stock (page 56) will neutralize nitrosamines.

Chicken Pâté

Chicken, lamb, beef, and other animals' livers are all nutrition powerhouses. Chicken liver is typically used in pâté recipes. It has more vitamin K2, D3, C, and iron than beef liver. This recipe is adapted from the article "Nourishing a Growing Baby" by Jenn Allbritton, C.N..

2 ounces (55 g) raw chicken liver

¼ cup (60 ml) Souper Stock (page 56)

1 to 2 teaspoons ghee

⅛ teaspoon Celtic sea salt

Add the liver to the stock. Bring the liquid to a boil and then reduce heat and simmer for 7 to 10 minutes. Remove from heat.

Purée the mixture together with the ghee. Thin with extra stock, mom's milk, or homemade formula (see chapter 8) to desired consistency.

Divide into 5 equal portions, resulting in about 10 grams of liver per serving (2 ounces liver equals approximately 55 grams); serve no more than once per day.

Yield: 2 servings

Note

- It's okay to freeze any leftovers.

Oh-So-Much-Better Than Cereal O's

Taking the Toxins Out

8 to 10 Months

This is an exciting time of beginning independence for your little one. Movement takes priority at this age. Your baby might get distracted during meals, as she might want to practice her new motor skills instead of sitting still to eat. Not to worry—she'll eat when she's hungry.

Part of your baby's exploration of the world is the practice of bringing everything to her mouth (and if empty-handed, her own dimpled fingers or toes will suffice). Though it's adorable, many parents are very concerned about how this behavior constantly exposes their babies to germs. Fortunately, most germs are helpful and shouldn't worry you. You would, however, be wise to be wary of *other* unseen dangers: the ubiquitous toxins in her food and environment. Recognizing toxins as the real health issues they are will help you take the necessary steps to protect your baby from them.

This chapter highlights the most harmful and most frequently encountered toxins in foods and your baby's environment. Additionally it provides guidance on how to minimize exposure and reduce toxins' effects on your baby's mind and body, which is the second pillar (purity) of Super Nutrition.

Toxins Take Stabs at Health

Many governing agencies are becoming increasingly concerned about the effects of dietary and environmental toxins on our children. Due to all the toxins that moms accumulate throughout their lives, 100 percent of babies are now *born* with a significant toxic load—before even taking their first breath of air. In fact, a 2004 study showed that the cord blood of newborns contained more than *200* industrial chemicals.

More toxins than ever! Chemicals in our food, water, and environment are on a sharp upswing, made especially worse with massive oil spills and nuclear power plant disasters; therefore, babies today face the greatest toxic burden ever known. Kenneth Bock, M.D., in *Healing the New Childhood Epidemics*, sums up the pollutants surrounding us:

▸ Drinking water: hydrocarbons, pathogens, and waste
▸ Air: mercury, lead, diesel exhaust, and other pollutants
▸ Oceans: poison, "especially mercury"
▸ Foods: chemicals, hormones, and antibiotics

Dr. Bock notes, "The total toxic burden on the average American [child] is measurably higher than it was even 10 years ago."

Our food supply has become polluted in many different ways, which is why it is so important to protect our children with optimal nutrition. Doing what you can to reduce toxins, while nourishing your baby as best as you can, will go far to help protect her from severe toxic attacks on her health.

SAD foods with toxic additives. Processed foods in the Standard American Diet (SAD) are dismantled, refined, bleached, and deodorized. They have stabilizers, emulsifiers, flavorings, colorings, thickeners, texturizers, and more. What nutrients they have are mostly synthetic and are poor replacements for the real thing. The FDA maintains a list of more than *3,000* additives that are part of our food supply (80 percent of which have not been tested for carcinogenic, immunotoxic, or neurotoxic effects).

Toxins from radiation-exposed foods. Meats, produce, and seasonings are typically irradiated (treated with radiation) to extend shelf life, in addition to having been exposed to environmental radiation. In studies, animals fed irradiated feed experienced early death, reproductive problems, cancer, chromosomal abnormalities, liver damage, and vitamin deficiencies.

Toxins from man-made DNA. *Seventy percent* of the foods consumed in the Standard American Diet are genetically modified, particularly corn and soy, but even *animals* are now undergoing genetic modification of their DNA. To force foreign DNA into the host, toxins, bacteria, and viruses are used. (For more on genetic modification, see page 149.)

Toxic SAD produce. Conventional farming today relies heavily on chemical pesticides, herbicides, fungicides, insecticides, and fertilizers. In fact, the USDA and FDA allow 275 pesticides to be sprayed on our produce, typically by workers wearing gas masks. If you serve a nonorganic apple to your baby, you are also serving up an average of sixteen pesticides applied at least thirty-six times.

Toxic SAD water. Municipal (or tap) water has purposefully added toxic chemicals like fluoride and chlorine, which kill friendly gut flora and disrupt metabolism. Though some pediatricians recommend fluoride supplements and fluoridated water for babies, newer research shows that fluoride is ineffective in protecting teeth and is actually harmful. (See "The Truth about Fluoride," page 71.) Other, unintentional chemicals and toxins are also present in water—lead, hormones, antibiotics, and rocket fuel to name just a few. Well water can contain chemicals that have leached into the ground or accumulated in rainwater, especially if the well is near a factory, golf course, or farm.

Toxic SAD animal foods. Regular farm animals have it very rough these days. They are fed genetically modified, mold-ridden, inflammatory, pesticide-treated, grain-based "feed." They are kept in giant overcrowded warehouses, rather than allowed to naturally graze outside. This unnatural diet and confinement-based lifestyle makes the animals so sickly that they require frequent antibiotics to keep them alive long enough to make it to market. Drugs, like steroids and growth hormone, are used to put extra weight on or to keep cows lactating. In fact, *70 percent* of big pharmaceutical companies' drug sales are made to our farm animals! In all, these animal foods are sources of toxins and drugs in our bodies, as well as inflammation and infection. They are also far less nutritious than animal foods from animals living their natural lifestyles and eating their natural diets. Animal foods from today's modern "farms" are very SAD, indeed.

Toxic SAD food packaging. Foods are abundantly packaged, stored, and heated in plastics. Some packaging is aseptic, killing even the beneficial bacteria that should exist in foods, while others, like most aluminum cans, contain chemicals such as bisphenol A (BPA), which is an endocrine disruptor and may lead to male feminization. These chemicals are often quite toxic to the human body. We urge you to reduce plastic food storage to whatever degree possible, opting for glass, stainless steel, or ceramic at every opportunity.

Combined and cumulative effects. Individual toxins are harmful enough on their own, yet they are *even more* harmful in combination. Today toxins travel in packs—it is rare to be exposed to just one at a time. In fact, so many exist that the possible combinations in which they can occur in foods, water, and the environment are too numerous to count or properly test. The few studies done, however, show that what one toxin could do alone is made much worse by the presence of another toxin—making the reality of combined and cumulative toxic effects today that much more worrisome.

The Truth about Fluoride

Fluoride, an industrial waste by-product that was once used to treat people with overactive thyroids, was added to municipal water supplies in an attempt to minimize dental decay. While the safety of fluoride has been questioned since the 1950s, no longer can the undeniable facts be ignored. Fluoride is toxic, especially to our bones, thyroids, and nervous systems.

Damages teeth and bones. According to Ruth Yaron, M.S., in *Super Baby Food*, 80 percent of American children have dental fluorosis (mottling and breakdown of the teeth) resulting from *too much* fluoride. Fluoride damage to teeth is an indicator of what is going on with bones. Yaron notes, "It is well known now that fluoride produces faulty bones, more brittle, basically mimicking in the bone what is clearly visible in the teeth."

Poisonous. All fluoride toothpastes have a warning to call Poison Control if swallowed. Fluoride is neurotoxic and damages more than 200 enzymes in the body. Further, according to David Brownstein, M.D., author of *Iodine: Why You Need It, Why You Can't Live Without It*, fluoride blocks iodine absorption, increasing the likelihood of thyroid disease and cancers. Iodine deficiency caused, in part, by too much fluoride, "is the most common preventable form of mental retardation known."

No help for decay. Some *might* consider all these adverse risks to be worth it if fluoride offered significant benefit to teeth, but fluoride has never actually been proven to prevent cavities! In fact, a study presented in 2010 by the American Chemical Society explains that the "protective layer" produced by topical fluoride is so thin that it is quickly worn away by ordinary chewing.

In January 2011, the U.S. Department of Health and Human Services finally lowered the maximum amount of fluoride allowed in water. This is just a slight improvement, as the safest measure would be to remove fluoride entirely from our water supply.

This 1956 ad reads, "It's written all over her face; what comes in glass tastes good. . . . You see, glass itself is so pure it just can't damage the taste and purity of what's inside. And glass is so convenient for storage and re-use." Though plastic containers that leach toxins into our foods were not widely in use then, it's clear that the sanctity of glass containers for protecting food was known.

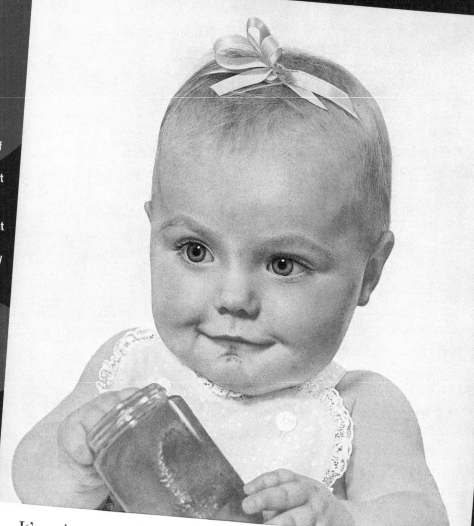

It's written all over her face; what comes in glass tastes good

And today, that's practically everything a baby eats. But baby isn't the only one learning to recognize the good flavor of food packed in glass. And good reason, too. You see, glass itself is so pure it just can't damage the taste and purity of what's inside. And glass is so convenient for storage and re-use. Ask your grocer for foods packaged in pure glass.

GLASS CONTAINER MANUFACTURERS INSTITUTE, 99 PARK AVENUE, NEW YORK

THE EFFECT OF THESE TOXINS ON BABIES IS THE 3C CONDITIONS!

Toxins in the body contribute to autism, asthma, allergies, learning disabilities like ADHD, and the other 3Cs. Experts from the National Institute of Environmental Health further report that even very low toxic exposure in early life is a factor in a variety of behavioral problems and autoimmune conditions.

For example, a study published in *Pediatrics*, the official journal of the American Academy of Pediatrics, reported on data from over one thousand children, showing that those with higher levels of organophophate-pesticides were twice as likely to have attention defecit hyperacticity disorder (ADHD).

Organophosphates belong to a class of pesticides that work by destroying the neurological systems of pests. They are neurotoxic in high doses so it isn't hard to imagine that they could also damage the brain-functioning of children. This class of pesticides has also been linked to childhood leukemia, lower IQs in children whose mothers were exposed to them, and is likely the cause of the destruction of the honeybee population (necessary to pollinate food crops).

Philip J. Landrigan, M.D., M.Sc., chair of the Department of Community Medicine at Mount Sinai School of Medicine and director of the Center for Children's Health and the Environment at Mount Sinai, provides several examples of toxins' causal role in disease. He states that asthma is exacerbated by air pollution; developmental delays are caused by lead in paint and contaminated drinking water; and pediatric cancers are caused by radiation and benzene.

When children can no longer handle the toxic burden, then one or more of the 3C conditions manifest. Depending on the child's inherent ability to handle the toxins, as well as to what particular cocktail of toxins she is exposed, the manifestation of toxic overload can be any of the 3Cs.

A Better Way to Reduce Toxins and Their Effects

Dr. Landrigan explains that the 3Cs (he calls them the "new pediatric morbidities") are of "toxic environmental origin," and therefore can *"be prevented* by reducing or eliminating children's exposures to toxic chemicals in the environment" and in the diet.

Environmental toxins. Take measures to research and reduce overall toxic exposure for your baby, paying attention to cleaning products, toys, bath soaps, sunscreens, lotions, clothing, and more. Ensure that soaps and products do not contain antibacterial agents such as triclosan (a toxic agent). Take shoes off when you enter your home (to avoid tracking in chemicals) and take great caution when your home is undergoing renovation. Refer to the chart on page 76 to see what could be toxic in your child's environment.

Vaccinations. Whether the benefits of vaccinations outweigh the risks is for parents to decide, but no one can disagree that there are toxins within vaccines. Although thimerosal (a preservative) is no longer used, it was replaced with other toxins such as aluminum (a neurotoxin) and formaldehyde (listed as a carcinogen in 2011 by the U.S. Department of Health and Human Services).

Vaccines and their toxins become more of a risk for under-nourished children. Nutrient deficiencies, particularly vitamin A, B12, and folic acid, can increase the risk of side effects from vaccinations, explains Russell L. Blaylock, M.D., neurosurgeon, nutrition researcher, excitotoxin expert, and author of in *Health and Nutrition Secrets*. He notes that vaccinating vitamin A–deficient African children and aboriginal populations in Australia "resulted in a very high mortality rate." Further, vitamin A, B12, and folic acid deficiencies increase the risk of a rare vaccination side effect that damages the brain and spinal cord. Providing your baby cod liver oil, liver, and butter regularly will ensure her levels of vitamin A, B12, and folic acid are sufficient for protection.

Minimize toxins in water. We recommend filtered, ideally reverse osmosis, water for all food and drink preparation for you and your baby. Since toxins in water can be absorbed through the skin, it would also be best to use filtered water to bathe your baby. (See Resources, page 218, for fixture-based filters.)

Minimize toxins in food. Choose organic produce as much as possible, particularly when consuming the foods that are the most pesticide contaminated. (See "The Dirty Dozen and the Clean Fifteen," page 78.) Wash all produce with a vegetable/fruit wash containing grapefruit seed extract to reduce the external pesticides and radiation. Animal fats store toxins, so by selecting organic meat or meat from grass-fed and pastured animals, you will be consuming the least toxins, pesticides, and heavy metals.

Since a major source of toxic exposure for children is through pesticide-ridden foods, particularly GMO foods, protective nutrition includes limiting conventional produce and animal foods and serving organic to your child as much as possible. By doing so, you can lower his risk for developing ADHD and other 3C conditions related to neurotoxicity like autism.

NUTRIENT-RICH SUPER POWER FOODS REDUCE TOXIC DAMAGE!

Nutrients and nutrient-rich foods can reduce toxic effects. Here are just a few examples from scientific research and medical studies:

▸ Antioxidants substantially protect against radiation.

▸ Iodine reduces thyroid cancer–causing effects of radiation exposure.

▸ Iodine sufficiency reduces the toxic effects of fluoride, chloride, and bromine and helps the body excrete heavy metals.

▸ Selenium renders mercury markedly less toxic.

▸ Molybdenum substantially decreases sensitivity to sulfites.

▸ Taurine protects the liver and testicles from toxic effects of cadmium.

▸ Vitamin B1 and molybdenum break down acetylaldehyde (which dulls the brain and is carcinogenic).

▸ Calcium, zinc, and essential vitamins reduce the toxic effects of lead and excess manganese.

▸ Saturated fatty acids protect the liver from medications.

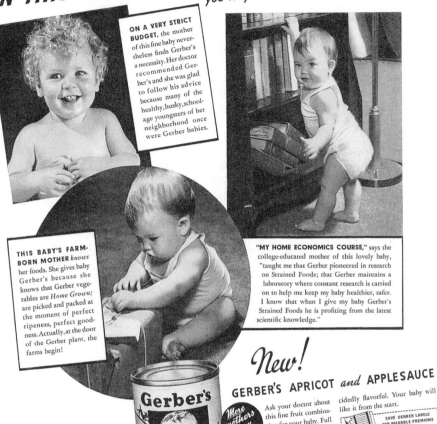

WE CAN'T SHOW YOU A MILLION BABIES ON THIS PAGE . . .
but let the Mothers of these three tell you Why More Mothers Buy Gerber's

ON A VERY STRICT BUDGET, the mother of this fine baby nevertheless finds Gerber's a necessity. Her doctor recommended Gerber's and she was glad to follow his advice because many of the healthy, husky, school-age youngsters of her neighborhood once were Gerber babies.

THIS BABY'S FARM-BORN MOTHER *knows* her foods. She gives baby Gerber's because she knows that Gerber vegetables are *Home Grown;* are picked and packed at the moment of perfect ripeness, perfect goodness. Actually, at the door of the Gerber plant, the farms begin!

"MY HOME ECONOMICS COURSE," says the college-educated mother of this lovely baby, "taught me that Gerber pioneered in research on Strained Foods; that Gerber maintains a laboratory where constant research is carried on to help me keep my baby healthier, safer. I know that when I give my baby Gerber's Strained Foods he is profiting from the latest scientific knowledge."

New!
GERBER'S APRICOT and APPLESAUCE

More mothers buy Gerber's

Ask your doctor about this fine fruit combination for your baby. Full ripe (not dried) apricots from the Santa Clara Valley of California and selected Michigan-grown apples, make a combination which not only supplies important vitamins and minerals — but which is de- cidedly flavorful. Your baby will like it from the start.

Gerber's STRAINED FOODS READY FOR USE

11 VARIETIES

The happy Gerber Baby on the blue and white label is your assurance of an honest product, made from selected ingredients of first quality, scientifically prepared to retain their vitamins and minerals to a high degree.

PEAS . . . BEETS . . . CEREAL . . . GREEN BEANS
VEGETABLE SOUP . . . TOMATOES . . . SPINACH
PRUNES . . . CARROTS
APRICOT AND APPLE SAUCE
LIVER SOUP WITH VEGETABLES

SAVE GERBER LABELS FOR VALUABLE PREMIUMS
Send for free, illustrated folder containing a variety of useful and valuable premiums given for Gerber labels and a few cents. Write your name and address on margin and send to Dept. 53.
GERBER PRODUCTS CO., FREMONT, MICH.
(In Canada, Gerber's are grown and packed by The Foods of Canada, Ltd., Tecumseh, Ontario.)

Common Sources of Environmental Toxins

Household Toxins	Food Additive Toxins
• Chlorine bleach • Chemical cleaners • Perfumes and fragrance • Building/construction materials and solvents • Fluoride • Fabric softeners • Petroleum jelly and mineral oil • Plastic/phthalates—store in glass instead • Cookware—nonstick and aluminum and microwave • Plastic toys • Vinyl and PVC toys and lunch boxes—also contain lead • Teethers with phthalates • Candles with lead wicks • Paints with VOCs—volatile organic compounds • Paint thinners • Adhesives • Fabric softener • Cigarette smoke • Styrofoam • Microwave ovens • Plastic water bottles, food storage containers, baby bottles • Teflon pans • Aluminum pans • Detergents and chemical cleaners • Antibacterial products: soaps, gels, cleansers, lunch boxes, diaper bags (triclosan) • Chlorine bleach • Water with chlorine, chloramine, fluoride, and/or lead • Lead in dishware, pipes, or paint • Carpeting • Wood products (plywood, chipboard) • Mildew and mold in home • Pesticide spraying • Arsenic-treated wood in playgrounds or desks (green-tinted) • New cars (dashboard, upholstery) • EMFs (electro-magnetic frequencies) • Dry cleaning • Bromine in furniture, electronics, mattresses • Asbestos • Formaldehyde • BPA (bisphenol A)	• Artifical sweeteners (aspartame, sucralose) and artificially sweetened foods • Nitrites and nitrates—bacon, hot dogs, sausage, bologna • Sulfites—lettuce, dried fruits, fresh fruits and vegetables (especially in restaurants), processed potato products, corn by-products • Sorbic acid—cheese, frosting, dried fruit, dips • Dyes (esp. yellow #5)—hundreds of processed, colored foods • Parabens—jelly, soda pop, pastry, beer, cake, salad dressing • Benzoic acid—soda pop, fruit juice, margarine, apple cider • Monosodium glutamate (MSG), also hydrolyzed vegetable protein and texturized vegetable protein—bouillon, Chinese restaurant dishes, chicken broth or flavoring; may also be in glutamate, sodium caseinate, calcium caseinate, or yeast extract • EDTA—margarine, salad dressing, frozen dinners, other processed foods • Propyl gallate—frozen dinners, gravy mix, turkey sausage • Alginate—ice cream, salad dressing, cheese spread, frozen dinners • Bromates—baked goods, bread crumbs, refrigerated dough • Growth hormone in foods

Hidden Toxins	Food Ingredient Toxins	Personal Care Toxins
• Heavy metals • Lead, cadmium, mercury, aluminum, arsenic; polluted air, water, soil, food • Lead in water supply from lead pipes • Aluminum-processed soy products, aluminum cookware, refined table salt, deodorants, antacids, baking powder, aluminum in vaccines • Mercury-amalgam fillings, linked to Alzheimer's and a number of other disease conditions **Unhealthy gut flora** • Toxins produced by yeast and fungus in the gut, such as ethanol and acetyldehyde • Toxins produced by pathogenic bacteria, such as sulfites (from sulphate-reducing pathogens) • Toxins created by incomplete protein digestion, such as gluteomorphin and casomorphin	• MSG (aka monosodium glutamate, hydrolyzed vegetable protein, hydrolyzed corn protein, autolyzed yeast, yeast extract/food, caseinate) • Colors and dyes • Preservatives • Flavorings • BHA and GHT • Annatto • Emulsifiers • Nitrates/nitrites • Sorbates • Sulfites • Table salt and baking powder with aluminum • Artificial flavors (like vanillin) • Trans fats (all hydrogenated oils—fully or partially) • Farm-raised fish with PCBs • Time-released pharmaceutical drugs • Mercury in fish • Aluminum cans, often lined with plastic • Antacids with aluminum • Fluoride tablets • Artificial sweeteners and fats • Nonorganic poultry and rice (may contain arsenic) • Genetically modified food • Chlorine in water • Fluoride in water and baby foods	• Deodorant with aluminum • Triclosan (antibacterial agent) • Synthetic fragrances • Nail polish • Soaps with parabens • Hairspray, hair gels, mousses with phthalates • Makeup with phthalates, lead, synthetic ingredients • Lice-killing products • Shampoos • Infant sleepwear and pajamas that are flame retardant (antimony) • Toothpaste with fluoride and artificial ingredients

Primary Source: *Nourishing Hope for Autism*, Julie Matthews

The Dirty Dozen and the Clean Fifteen

It's hard to afford organic 100 percent of the time, so here we provide a list of foods, compiled by the Environmental Working Group, that should always be purchased organic, and a list that can be consumed nonorganic to meet budgetary constraints. (For a full list of forty-nine fruits and vegetables, and where they rank in terms of pesticide contamination, visit the Environmental Working Group's website, www.foodnews.org.)

The Dirty Dozen

The most contaminated foods come first.

1. Celery
2. Peaches
3. Strawberries
4. Apples
5. Blueberries (domestic)
6. Nectarines
7. Sweet bell peppers
8. Spinach
9. Cherries
10. Kale/collard greens
11. Potatoes
12. Grapes (imported)

The Clean Fifteen

These foods, the most "clean" coming first, have the lowest pesticide load.

1. Onions
2. Avocado
3. Sweet corn (frozen; while low in pesticides, still has risk of GMO)
4. Pineapples
5. Mango (subtropical and tropical)
6. Sweet peas (frozen)
7. Asparagus
8. Kiwi fruit (subtropical and tropical)
9. Cabbage
10. Eggplant
11. Cantaloupe (domestic)
12. Watermelon
13. Grapefruit
14. Sweet potatoes
15. Honeydew melon

Antioxidants help disarm toxins. They are necessary to prevent and reduce the consequences of toxins, such as brain damage and inflammation, both of which make organs and systems unable to function normally (leading to disease). According to Elizabeth Lipski, Ph.D., C.C.N., clinical nutritionist and author of *Digestive Wellness for Children*, "the average person is exposed to over 100 different chemicals [every day]. If we get enough antioxidants . . . from our foods, we can easily slough off most chemical toxins."

Fruits, vegetables, and greens contain important antioxidants such as vitamin C and bioflavonoids, but you might be surprised to learn that *animal foods* contain many key antioxidants and the raw "materials" (nutrients) for synthesizing more!

Further, eating probiotic-rich foods and probiotic supplements reduce the amount of toxins that can gain access to your baby's bloodstream through his intestinal wall. When probiotic protection is adequate, heavy metals and other toxins are blocked to by the probiotics, thus kept out of the blood, and will be excreted in the stool.

As Robert Bernadini points out in *The Truth About Children's Health,* "The amount of . . . [toxins] that wouldn't harm well-nourished individuals may *poison undernourished* children." If you provide your baby with a diet based on Super Nutrition, toxins they're exposed to will be far less damaging.

Common Baby Food Pitfalls

Taking measures to reduce toxins for your baby means including more nutritious dietary options. By simply making better-than-average choices regarding beverages and finger foods at this age, you'll go far to protect your baby's health.

JUICE IS JUST AN ILLUSION OF HEALTHFULNESS

Despite having no nutritional benefits and consistent recommendations to limit it, juice remains a socially acceptable drink for babies, toddlers, and kids. Unfortunately, the AAP reports that almost 90 percent of infants under one year of age are given juice—and some are consuming more than 16 ounces (475 ml) per day!

Store-bought *juice is naught more than sugar water*, or "liquid candy." (Unfortunately, organic, 100 percent juice isn't any better because it is still mostly sugar, lacking the fiber, enzymes, and nutrients of whole fruit.) Juice is bad for your baby because it disrupts her health in several ways.

Juice displaces nutrient-rich foods. Babies often get full from juice such that they are no longer hungry for nutritious food and drink. Moreover, the *addicting* nature of juice means that children will keep asking for it.

Juice is an impetus for tooth decay. No one can dispute the role that juice and sweetened drinks play in the development of tooth decay. The AAP advises that babies "should not be given juice from bottles or easily transportable covered cups that allow them to consume juice easily throughout the day."

Juice weakens immunity. Studies show that sugar in juice reduces immune function by disabling critical white blood cells for five to seven hours after ingestion, which makes them less able to fight off infection. The immune system is effectively "stunned" by sugar, fructose, honey, and even *100 percent* juice.

Juice causes bellyaches and diarrhea. The AAP warns that excessive juice consumption can be associated with diarrhea, flatulence, and abdominal distention and can lead to malnutrition. In *My Tummy Hurts*, Joseph Levy, M.D., warns that "juice abuse" *causes* diarrhea and likely promotes obesity.

Juice is a source of heavy metals. If all that isn't enough to discourage you from giving your baby juice, in 2010, a California study found that 80 percent of all juice (yes, organic too) contains the dangerous toxin *lead*! And since 40 percent of high fructose corn syrup (HFCS) samples contain mercury, juice made with HFCS is likely to contain harmful *mercury* as well.

We recommend only filtered water as an additional, but not required, beverage at this age. Offer water to your baby especially when it is hot outside and others are thirsty. If you feel your baby is ready to try using a cup, Souper Stock (page 56) is another acceptable beverage in small quantities.

FINGER FOODS TO FORGO

Cereal (like Cheerios) is the most common finger food babies eat to practice their pincer grasp. Moms typically throw a plastic container or bag full of such cereal into their diaper bags to have at a moment's notice. Teething crackers, biscuits, and cookies are also commonplace in the diets of babies, starting at this age.

While cereals remain an expected finger food, surprisingly, there is little rationale for giving them. In fact, cereal proves to be a harmful CRAP food!

Chemical:

Processed grain products are a source of toxins. Due to the processing they endure, cereals are sources of toxins. Cereals (and most teething crackers) are created via a high-heat process called extrusion, which denatures proteins, turning them into neurotoxins. Whole grains are even worse, as they contain more protein. Further, extrusion damages fatty acids and even destroys many added vitamins and minerals.

Grains Take a Toxic Turn When Turned into Cereal

The Weston A. Price Foundation notes unpublished studies that show the toxicity of extruded grains (like breakfast cereal). In one case, rats eating just the cereal box lived longer than those eating the cereal! In another study, using puffed wheat cereal, rats fed the cereal and fortified water died in just 1 month, much sooner than the rats who were fed *only* water. This is likely due to toxins in the cereal.

Due to high heat during processing, cereals also contain more than 500 times the safe limit of a class 2A toxin: acrylamides. This toxin causes cancer and has a variety of other toxic effects in human and animal studies. A popular finger-food cereal for babies ranks second highest in the top ten acrylamide offenders. Studies further show that the lower the nutrient content of the grains, the higher the amount of acrylamide created during processing.

Removes body's nutrients:

Cereal is sugar loaded. Even "healthy" cereals contain some form of sugar; most contain many sources. Since the body uses nutrients to metabolize it, sugar—offering *no* nutrients—effectively steals nutrients from the body. While the box's label might look nutritious, cereal is more likely to deplete your child's body of nutrients than to supply them.

Grains are hard to digest. At this age, your baby is barely making the starch-digesting enzymes needed to digest grains (refer back to chapter 2). Gluten, a protein found in wheat, barley, rye, oats, and most cereals, is particularly hard to digest. Undigested proteins increase your child's risk of developing gluten intolerance and allergies.

Grain foods lead to autoimmune diseases. Early gluten introduction has been shown to play a role in the development of celiac disease, as well as other autoimmune disorders. Celiac disease occurs when the body reacts to gluten that isn't completely digested and causes an immune attack against not only undigested gluten but also intestinal tissue. As the incidence of celiac disease (and other autoimmune disorders) is on a steep rise, some experts postulate that this increase might be directly related to early and excessive gluten-containing diets, including an increasing reliance on grain foods for babies.

Addictive:

Cereals are a source of dietary opiates. A special enzyme (called DPP-4) is needed to digest gluten. Since babies don't yet have this gluten-busting enzyme, the gluten can get "stuck" in a partially digested form. Called gluteo*morphin*, this partially digested protein acts similar to other opiates—opium, morphine, and heroin—clouding and fogging the brain, hindering development and perception, and altering behavior. Since gluteomorphins *are just as addicting as other opiate drugs*, your baby can get physically hooked on cereal and wheat.

When eating cereal with pasteurized milk, another potential dietary opiate enters the mix. Just like poorly digested wheat can lead to gluteomorphins, a lack of DPP-4 can also lead to poorly digested casein from the milk, which results in casein*morphins* (other dietary opiates). For many children, having cereal with pasteurized milk delivers a double-whammy opiate effect.

Souper Stock and fermented foods increase stomach acidity and thus stimulate digestive enzymes, like DPP-4. Also, the gelatin in Souper Stock eventually *increases* the amount and activity of enzymes that break down gluteomorphin and caseomorphin. Feeding your baby Souper Stock (and cultured foods) will pay off when grains are finally introduced—he'll be better able to fully break down potential dietary opiates into their "kinder" amino acid building blocks. *Limiting toxins* will further help, since toxins deactivate these important enzymes.

Processed:

Processed, refined grains. Flour used in cereals is most often refined, meaning the whole grain is broken apart, the nutrient-rich portions removed and then it's "fortified" with *synthetic* vitamins and minerals, additional sugar, and flavorings.

The toxic, depleting, inflammatory, allergenic, and addictive nature of breakfast cereals make them a very *poor* choice for babies, as well as for children and adults. Can you do better than "O's" for your baby? Absolutely!

For preferable finger foods, refer to the recipes that begin on page 87.

Safeguard Your Child against Toxins with Optimal Nourishment

We know toxins are everywhere, and they're bombarding your baby at every turn! But, you *can* do something to help! *Toxins are not as damaging to well-nourished children*. If you provide your child with a diet based on Super Nutrition, she will not develop the 3C conditions as readily as undernourished, nutrient-depleted babies and children.

WHAT YOU CAN EXPECT AT THIS AGE

Self-feeding. Between 8 and 10 months, your baby will develop the "pincer grasp," which means touching an opposing finger together with his thumb, allowing him to grasp smaller objects. It is now time for some finger-friendly foods, giving your baby a chance to practice this

Super Nutrition Food Categorizations for 8 to 10 Months

Super POWER	PURE
Fish roe	Organic fruits
Raw yogurt or kefir	Organic vegetables
Raw butter	Organic pastured meats
Grass-fed, organic heart and liver	Organic coconut milk
Lacto-fermented veggies, roots, and fruits	Organic yogurt and kefir
Organic animal fats	Organic butter
	Organic eggs

OKAY	CRAP
Organic baby food (stage 2 to 3)	Breakfast cereal
Nonorganic, non–Dirty Dozen fruits and vegetables, washed	Prepackaged "baby" meals
All-natural meats	Teething biscuits, crackers, cookies
Nonorganic butter	Baby food with added sugar, juice, fruit concentrate, or anything other than fruit, vegetable, or meat
	Juice (organic or nonorganic)

new grip and become more confident with self-feeding. Even if your baby isn't yet interested in feeding himself, let him play and explore and get used to holding an extra spoon as well as touching, feeling, even squishing foods.

More texture. Part of digestion is the mechanical breakdown of foods by chewing. Even though your baby may not have teeth yet, his hard gums can mash foods, and he is now capable of eating more textured foods. At 8 months, food purées and mashes should be thicker than they have been so far, with very soft, squishy lumps; less mom's milk or homemade/enriched formula is needed for thinning. By 9 months, foods should be chunkier, though chunks should still be soft and smooshy. Once babies can

tolerate these chunkier foods well, without choking (usually around 9 months), it is time to consider adding finger foods.

How much? By 8 months, meal sizes will still vary based on your baby's hunger and nutrient needs, but on average will consist of one to four tablespoons (15 to 55 g) of a food (which is 1/4 cup [55 g], or two frozen cubes). Some babies will be hungry enough at a meal to consume 1/2 cup (115 g) of food. Follow your baby's hunger signs and stop feeding when she becomes no longer interested or turns her head to the side when you move the spoon toward her.

Continue nursing about five times per day, or give 25 to 32 ounces (700 to 950 ml) of formula in 24 hours. By 9 months, meals become more important to satisfy nutritional needs, though nursing and bottles are still important for complete nutrition, comfort, bonding, and to satisfy your baby's suckling instinct. If your baby is not interested much in food, you may need to reduce the quantity of mom's milk or formula.

How many foods per meal? During this age, meals will start to be made up of more than one food. Always serve an animal protein or fat with each meal. New foods should be accompanied by already-introduced foods. That way, any adverse reactions will be recognized as from the new food. Continue to introduce new foods every 3 to 4 days.

Recipes to Help Protect Against Toxins

Between the ages of 8 and 10 months, nutrient needs remain ever critical. Requirements for absorbable iron, zinc, and copper are still high. Protein needs are not quite half met through nursing or formula intake, so animal foods continue to be a very important part of your baby's diet. For a more complete list of acceptable foods at this age, see the Food Introduction Timeline on page 222.

FEEDING AT 8 MONTHS

At around 8 months of age, you can start introducing gelatin, fish roe, some new veggies, a few tree fruits, and a wide variety of meats cooked in Souper Stock (page 56). Continue to include the nutritious and digestible meals introduced for 6- and 7-month-olds in your baby's diet. Recall that nutrients work to protect against toxins, so the nutrient-dense food suggestions that follow will serve to protect your child and are sufficiently pure so as not to add to her toxic burden, either.

Meals usually continue at twice per day until 9 months. Often, meals are still accompanied by nursing or bottles or are fit in between feedings. The following chart shows the feeding pattern we suggest.

Pattern	8 months
Early AM	Milk / homemade formula
Mid-Morning	Milk / homemade formula + snack
Mid-Day	Milk (new food every 3 to 4 days)
Afternoon	Milk / homemade formula
Evening	Meal
Nighttime	Milk / homemade formula

Finger-Fun Gelatin Jigglers

Store-brand instant-gelatin dessert is a source of various toxins: The gelatin is exposed to bleach; artificial colorings and dyes are used to color it; and it contains 19 grams of sugar or artificial sweeteners per quarter package. (Sugar-free gelatin is also highly processed and contains artificial sweeteners, which are themselves a source of toxins.) Unprocessed gelatin, however, is pure, provides important amino acids, and is a bonus gift to the digestive tract.

Pears or apples, peeled and cored

2¹/₂ tablespoons (18 g) Bernard Jensen's gelatin (www.radiantlifecatalog.com)

Use a Vitamix blender or juicer to make fresh juice from whole fruit. Two pears or apples will equal 2¹/₃ cups (555 ml) juice. Simmer the juice, minus ¹/₂ cup (120 ml), in a saucepan over medium heat.

If you don't own a juicer, heat the fruit in a saucepan over medium-low heat, stirring occasionally, until liquefied, about 1 hour. (McIntosh apples break down the fastest.) Purée the apples or pears with an immersion blender, if needed. (Have caution when blending hot liquids.) Set aside 2¹/₃ cups (555 ml), cooling ¹/₂ cup (120 ml).

Sprinkle the gelatin evenly over the ¹/₂ cup (120 ml) cool liquid. Set aside for 10 minutes until the gelatin has absorbed the liquid. (If it's not fully absorbed, gently stir to combine.)

Add the gelatin mixture to the hot fruit liquid, stirring in slowly and consistently to ensure the gelatin fully dissolves.

Pour into an 8 × 8-inch (20 × 20 cm) glass baking dish or (other shallow glass container) and refrigerate for at least 3 hours.

Slice into small finger-fun for your baby.

Yield: 64 one-inch (2.5 cm) cubes

Notes

- Tropical fruits cannot be used to make gelatin; because they are so enzyme rich, their busy digestive activity will break down (predigest) the gelatin and it will never "set."
- We do not recommend using store-bought juice (see discussion on juice, page 79). For an even less-sweet version, substitute 1 cup (235 ml) of the homemade fruit juice with filtered water.
- Use apples or pears (peeled for 8-month-olds), and introduce berries at 10 to 12 months. After 1 year, try juicing well-cooked greens to infuse some veggie nutrition into the jigglers.

Baby "Caviar" Has Super POWERs

Not just for yachts and villas, caviar has "billion-dollar" benefits your baby can enjoy. In fact, fish roe is an ancient sacred food for preconception, pregnancy, nursing moms, and growing children.

Fish roe's small size, shape, and stickiness make them fun practice for the pincer grasp. These nutrient-rich eggs have vitamin A, K2, zinc, iodine, DHA and are a very rich source of vitamin D. (If you're giving your baby additional vitamin D or are taking it yourself, you can skip your dose on the days you both consume roe. Some studies show one tablespoon of fish eggs contains 17,000 IU of precious vitamin D.)

In fact, *fish roe is a Super POWER food*:

P—Protective—builds the brain, supports the immune system and digestive health

O—Optimal nutrition—very nutrient dense

W—Wisdom of the ancients—a traditional food around the world

E—Enriching—mineral and vitamin rich, especially with vitamin D

R—Regenerating—a healing food, used for fertility and for growing optimally healthy babies

Fancy Fish Roe

Fish roe (eggs) are Super POWER foods for your baby. She will be fascinated chasing them around her high-chair tray. They are great for trying out her new pinching-style grasp and bringing them to her mouth as self-feeding practice. While most fish are contaminated with heavy metals, fish eggs are the cleanest "fish" you can get. This Super POWER food packs a powerful punch for protection against toxins.

1 teaspoon fish roe (raw, frozen, or dried)

Coconut oil or ghee (see "Fabulous Fats," page 176), optional

Fresh fish roe usually requires no preparation. If frozen, just thaw it. Some roe might require removing casings.

Warm the roe in a pan lightly coated with coconut oil or ghee, if desired.

1 teaspoon is a good serving size for self-feeding, but the roe can also be stirred into a soft-boiled egg yolk (page 55), mixed with mashed avocado, stirred into Souper Stock meat meals (page 88), or served together with puréed vegetables.

Yield: 1 serving

Notes
- Purchase only refrigerated roe, as shelf-stable caviar contains preservatives, or order online.
- Salmon roe is largest and best for first finger foods.
- Avoid domestic paddlefish caviar from the contaminated rivers of Mississippi, Ohio, and Tennessee.

Veggie Varietal: Zucchini, Parsnips, and Celery

Carrots, squash, and sweet potatoes are often the first veggies we think of for our babies. While greens and raw and salad vegetables aren't yet appropriate for your baby's digestive system, a few other options can widen her palate and increase nutrients. How about zucchini, parsnips, and celery? These antioxidant- and nutrient-rich veggies will help enrich her immune and detoxification systems against toxins. (Make sure the celery is organic, as it's #1 on the Dirty Dozen list, page 78.)

1 zucchini, diced

3 parsnips, diced

2 stalks celery, diced

Souper Stock (page 56), optional

2 tablespoons (28 ml) olive oil; or use (28 g) coconut oil, red palm oil, ghee, butter, or (26 g) lard (see "Fabulous Fats," page 176), optional

To cook the the zucchini, parsnips, and celery, either sauté them in fat, steam, or simmer for 20 to 25 minutes in the stock until very soft. Remove the vegetables from the stock and mix with olive oil, coconut oil, red palm oil, ghee, butter, or lard and a pinch of high-quality Celtic sea salt.

After steaming, sautéing, or simmering, purée the veggies, thinning with more stock, mom's milk, or formula, as needed.

Yield: About 1½ cups (340 g) cooked veggies

Fantastic Finger Foods for 9 Months Plus

Below are great ideas for easy, quick, and nutritious finger foods:

- Fish roe
- Finger-Fun Gelatin Jigglers (page 85)
- Very soft, well-cooked carrots, rutabagas, or parsnips cut into very small chunks cooked in Souper Stock
- Very, very ripe peeled pear or peach chunks
- Baked sweet potato mashed with butter and rolled into easy-to-pick-up balls
- Chunks of soft avocado
- Chunks of very ripe banana
- Diced small, stewed apples or pears
- Very ripe and soft cantaloupe, mango, or papaya chunks, slightly mashed

Note
- Celery is very fibrous and should be extremely soft when served to your baby, which is why cooking for a long time in soup is recommended.

More Magnificent Meats and Souper Stock

Once you've mastered lamb, beef, and chicken, you can turn to turkey, bison, rabbit, pheasant, venison, duck, game hens, quail, goose, and pork as alternatives in the meat and broth meals, as they are also nutritious for your baby. Meats contain powerful antioxidants (namely carnosine, carnitine, and taurine), which protect the body and reduce toxins' damaging effects.

1 to 2 pounds (455 to 910 g) meat of your choice, cut into cubes

1 recipe Souper Stock (page 56)

2 cups (about 220 g) acceptable veggies for baby at this age, optional

Cook the meat in the stock. After cooking, cool the meat and then purée a serving size for your baby.

Thin to desired texture with more Souper Stock, mom's milk, or formula. You may also add the veggies from the stock, as well as fats (including coconut oil, ghee, butter, or olive oil) to the purées.

Optional: Meats can also be roasted in the oven but should still be puréed with the stock to aid digestion.

Yield: 4 servings for baby and a meal-sharing adult

Note

- Choose meats that are pastured (grass fed) from organic sources (try www.uswellnessmeats.com or a local pastured farm co-op near you).

Mom to Mom / Look at the stickers on produce. A five-digit number beginning with 9 is organic. A five-digit number starting with an 8 is a GMO food. A four-digit number is a conventionally grown food—neither organic nor GMO. In terms of toxic pesticide exposure, this translates to:

- 9####—Organic: no or low pesticides, better nutrition, sustainable farming practices
- ####—Conventional: "normal" use of pesticides (varies based on food, see list, page 78)
- 8####—GMO: the most pesticides and all the risks of GMO (see page 149 for more about GMO)

Cherries, Apples, and Pears, Oh My!

One of the favors beneficial bacteria does for us is digest and break down fiber and other carbohydrates. Eventually your baby will have built up her army of beneficial bacteria, but until then, most vegetables and fruits should be cooked before serving to make them more digestible and nutritious—and therefore protective against toxins. As cherries, apples, and pears are within the top twenty most pesticide-ridden foods (see "The Dirty Dozen and the Clean Fifteen," page 78), choose organic, if possible. (If organic is not available, wash well with a natural wash containing grapefruit seed extract.) Peel, core, and chop pears and apples; pit cherries. Sauté the fruit with ghee or coconut oil over low heat until very soft or alternatively, simmer 1/2 cup (about 60 g) chopped fruit in 1 cup (235 ml) filtered water until very soft. Purée (use caution when puréeing hot liquids) and then thin to desired consistency with mom's milk or homemade formula. Cool and serve. Consider mixing the fruits with meats for new flavors.

Lacto-Fermented Fruit "Chutney"

Turning fruits into a lacto-fermented chutney enhances the nutrition, digestibility, and protective qualities of fruits and makes them a source of probiotics and vitamin K2! This recipe is adapted from Nourishing Traditions *by Sally Fallon.*

1 cup (about 125 g) finely chopped fruit (peeled apples, cherries, or pears)

Grated rind and juice of 1/4 orange

3 to 4 teaspoons (15 to 20 ml) Homemade Whey (page 64)

1/2 teaspoon Celtic sea salt

3 tablespoons (45 ml) filtered water

Mix all the ingredients and mash down into a mason jar. The liquid should cover the fruit. Cover tightly and leave at room temperature for 48 hours; then refrigerate.

Yield: About 1 cup (250 g)

Note

• Scoop out a serving size of about 2 tablespoons (16 g) to 1/4 cup (65 g) and purée. Serve with cooked meat dishes as a nutritious, delicious digestive aid.

FEEDING AT 9 MONTHS

By the time your baby is around 9 months old, meals will usually progress to three times per day. They may now be made of multiple foods and aren't always accompanied by formula or nursing. The following chart shows the feeding pattern we suggest.

Pattern	9 months
Early AM	Milk / homemade formula
Mid-Morning	Bottle or nursing and small meal
Mid-Day	Meal
Afternoon	Milk / homemade formula
Evening	Meal
Nighttime	Milk / homemade formula

"Heart"y Stew

Despite the popularity of lean muscle meats like chicken breast, certain beef cuts, and fish, rarely are heart or tongue consumed, though both are lean muscle meats. Traditional Peruvian, Chinese, Italian, English, and Hungarian cuisines include fabulous dishes with heart.

It is interesting that organ meats contain the nutrients that best feed that organ. Dietary heart is an excellent source of carnitine, taurine, B vitamins, and the antioxidant CoQ10, all of which individually show remarkable cardiovascular benefits, as well as neutralize the toxic damage of free radicals (found in environmental toxins, secondhand smoke, and other pollutants). Further studies that have looked at combining these nutrients have stunned researchers with their heart-health benefits.

½ medium onion, finely chopped

2 tablespoons (28 g) butter, ghee, coconut oil, or (26 g) lard

½ pound (225 g) beef heart, minced

½ pound (225 g) ground beef, optional

2 ounces (55 g) beef liver, optional

2 medium carrots, sliced

½ to 1 teaspoon Celtic sea salt

2½ cups (570 ml) Souper Stock (page 56)

Brown the onion in the fat over medium-high heat.

Lower the heat to medium and add the beef (along with the ground beef and liver, if using). Cook until brown. Add the carrots and sea salt and cook until the carrots are soft.

Fill the pan with enough stock (or filtered water if stock is not available) to cover the meat. Lower the heat to low, cover the pan, and simmer until the meat is very tender, about 2 to 3 hours.

Purée the meat with the vegetables and stock or cut the meat into very tiny bites and serve with stock.

Yield: Dinner for family, or 3 servings for baby and accompanying adult

Notes

- If you've served beef before, introducing well-cooked onions and heart at the same time is fine since heart is also beef muscle meat.
- Alternatively, you can simmer chopped heart overnight in a slow cooker of Souper Stock, with carrots, celery, and onion, along with a pinch of Celtic sea salt, marrow bones, and small bit of vinegar
- Additional seasonings like pepper and tarragon can be added at age one.

Butter

Butter—the best quality you can get*—is an important factor in Super Nutrition. It helps with proper metabolism, growth, and development as well as protects against heart disease, cancer, infection, arthritis, osteoporosis, and digestive problems. (For more on butter's benefits, see page 177.) *The more you can use this healthy food in your baby's diet—the better!*

*The best butter is unpasteurized, grass fed, and comes from a trusted raw-dairy farm. Next best is organic, pastured (grass-fed) butter.

Puréed Peaches and Apricots

This dish makes a great "dessert" or celebration "treat" for baby. There is no need to try a taste of ice cream or cake, which is harmful even in small quantities at this age—especially when Nature provides abundant flavor and natural sweetness as is found in apricots and peaches! Serving with enzyme- and probiotic-rich yogurt or plain, whole (preferably raw) kefir is delicious and will also help digestion.

2 peaches, peeled, pitted, and chopped
3 apricots, peeled, pitted, and chopped
Ghee or coconut oil

Cook the fruit in the fat over low heat until very soft.

Purée and thin a serving of 2 tablespoons (28 ml) to ¼ cup (60 ml) to desired consistency with mom's milk or homemade formula. Alternatively, bring ½ cup (85 g) chopped fruit to a boil in 1 cup (235 ml) filtered water. Reduce heat and simmer for 15 minutes.

Purée with the liquid (use caution when puréeing hot liquids), cool, and serve.

Optional: Thin the apricot or peach purée with unsweetened coconut milk to add interesting flavor and healthful fatty acids (particularly lauric acid, a potent antiviral fat found uniquely in mom's milk and coconut).

Yield: 1½ cups (384 g) (or about 6 baby servings)

Note
• Peaches are often high in pesticides. Choose organic if possible.

Yogurt and Kefir

Milk that has been cultured is a good source of protein, as well as vitamins, minerals, and probiotics. Fermented dairy provides *phenomenal* health benefits, such as improving calcium absorption, boosting immunity, aiding digestion and detoxification, and helping prevent and treat constipation, thrush, and yeast diaper rashes. Yogurt is fermented (curdled) milk. Kefir is similar to yogurt, but it's usually more liquid and has different microflora strains, including good yeast.

• *Raw* yogurt and kefir are vastly preferred. (Check with local CSAs and farm co-ops.)
• Commercial yogurt should say "live" and "active" cultures so that the beneficial bacteria is living—which is the only way it does you any good. If the label says "pasteurized," "stabilized," or "heat-treated after culturing," then the bacteria will have all been destroyed by the heat processing. See Resources for recommended brands.
• Choose whole-milk, unflavored yogurt, as fats make the probiotics hardier and healthier, and flavors usually have added sugar.

Yogurt Cheese

Another way to get the benefits of cultured dairy is to strain the whey out of the yogurt and use the curds as a nutrient-rich "cream cheese."

2 cups (16 ounces, or 455 g) whole, plain, organic yogurt (preferably raw)

Let the sealed yogurt sit out on the counter for 24 hours. It will separate into whey (the yellow liquid) and milk solids (curds).

Line a mesh strainer with several layers of cheesecloth (or a coffee filter) and set over a bowl. Pour the yogurt in.

Let the whey drip through the strainer for 24 hours (remaining on the counter if raw dairy is used and in the refrigerator if using pasteurized dairy); the curds will be captured in the cloth. (If you suspend the strainer higher over the bowl, you'll make a "dryer" cheese.) This resulting yogurt cheese will be similar to cream cheese in consistency.

Mix with very soft fruits or vegetables.

Yield: About 1½ cups (12 ounces, or 340 g) "cheese"

Note
• Yogurt cheese will last 2 weeks in the refrigerator.

Little Green Trees and Purple Bushes

Broccoli is one of the most nutritious vegetables with anticancerous indoles, antioxidants, vitamins and minerals, and antidiabetic chromium. Cauliflower is a serious cancer fighter and has the energy-boosting B vitamin biotin. Look for cauliflower in a fun purple shade, which contains more toxin-protecting carotenes. Boiling neutralizes goitrogens naturally found in broccoli and cauliflower. Goitrogens block the production of thyroid hormone, which could lead to chills and "slow metabolism." The longer boiled, the greater the goitrogen reduction. However, limit broccoli and cauliflower consumption to once a week if your baby has congenital hypothyroidism or a significant family history of thyroid disorders. Boil the broccoli and cauliflower, separately, in water for 20 to 30 minutes until very soft. They should mash easily with a fork. Mix in ghee, butter, marrow, or other fabulous fat of your choice.

Fruits of the Tropics

Fruits such as passion fruit, guava, papaya, pineapple, kiwi, and cantaloupe are enzyme rich and when ripe are essentially predigested for your baby. Predigested foods tax the pancreas less, allowing certain enzymes to serve the immune cells better and faster. Peel and chop fresh fruits into small pieces for finger food. Or slightly mash them, depending on your baby's readiness. Pineapple is very sweet and should not be given too often nor in large quantities. With kiwi, cut out the white central core, as this may reduce oral irritation that some people experience.

Coconut Isn't a Nut, But a Healthy Palm Fruit

Though it contains the word *nut*, coconut is not part of the tree nut family or the legume family. Coconuts belong to the palm family, and allergies to coconut are very rare. Lab experts and allergists agree that nut allergies and coconut allergies are not related.

Coconut oil's benefits to health are many (see "Fabulous Fats," page 176). Copra, or coconut "meat," is a great source of fiber. Often called "nature's sports drink," coconut water is an excellent electrolyte solution. Coconut milk, as well, is very nutritious, offering minerals, vitamins, amino acids, and healthy fatty acids. In some cultures, it is a first food for babies starting at 6 months.

Coconut Custard

At around 9 months, fully cooked egg yolks can occasionally be used (despite enzymes being destroyed), as in this wonderful custard recipe. Coconut contains lauric acid, which is also found in mom's milk; the body uses lauric acid to make a very powerful antiviral agent in the body: monolaurin. Since the immune system and detoxification system often work hand-in-hand, strengthening one (with enzymes, antioxidants, vitamins, and minerals) will also help the other.

1 cup (235 ml) organic, whole coconut milk (with only guar gum added)

¹/₂ cup (112 g) softened or melted and cooled butter or ghee

¹/₂ brown-spotted banana, mashed

6 large egg yolks

Preheat the oven to 325°F (170°C, gas mark 3).

Mix all the ingredients until well combined. Pour the mixture into 8 buttered paper cups set in a muffin tin. Place the muffin tin in a 9 × 13-inch (23 × 33 cm) pan that has been filled two-thirds to three-quarters full with water. Bake for 45 minutes or until set.

Yield: 8 "muffin"-size custard cups

Notes
- Custards may be stored in the refrigerator for up to 5 days.
- As cans may be lined with BPA and refrigerated coconut milk often contains toxins like carrageenan, consider making your own coconut milk: Separate the brown outer portion of the coconut from the copra (meat). Roughly chop the copra and put in a blender with 1 cup (235 ml) hot water for every cup of copra. Blend and then strain the milk through cheesecloth.

4

Reconsider Baby Food Jars and Noodle Stars

Bolstering Immunity with Nutrients and Foods

10 to 12 Months

For a few months now you've been cautiously introducing foods at a slow pace, making sure the consistency is specific to what can be mashed between your baby's gums. Now you can work through new flavors faster and can relax a bit in terms of foods' consistency. Along with new foods, your baby will be putting everything else he can get his little hands on into his mouth. While that's fine most of the time, you will need to consider raising his defenses against potential illnesses.

Going to music, play-gym, or other "baby classes" might become part of your schedule. Such social excursions come with increased exposure to bacteria and viruses. While such exposure is important for your baby's developing immune system, it is important to fortify your baby with powerful immune-boosting foods to ensure that he has everything he needs to win the battles against those infectious agents. This is the hallmark of the third pillar (immune boosting) of Super Nutrition.

True Culprits of Illness

A typical illness-prevention tip advises avoiding microbes through disinfecting. Doctors, the media, and the Centers for Disease Control and Prevention (CDC) recommend frequent hand washing and the use of antibacterial soaps and hand-sanitizing gels as the *best* methods to avoid getting sick.

Yet we are constantly exposed to germs. But simply being exposed to a germ doesn't mean your baby will get sick. *Whether he gets sick is based on the strength of his immune system, not germ exposure alone.* In fact, the vast majority of bacteria are helpful. Ultimately, microbial exposure serves to strengthen immunity by *helping* your baby's gut develop and creates a strong barrier against agents that could make him sick. When he builds an army of good bacteria, they'll help him fight back.

A weak immune system is the true culprit behind illness. Struggling immunity comes from poor diet, sugar, toxins, antibiotic overuse, nutrient deficiencies, low omega-3 and high omega-6 fatty acids, protein deficiency, and lack of good bacteria.

The outsourcing of our immune system. With antibiotics being such a "quick fix," we've forgotten the importance of strengthening and fortifying our natural immune system. But with new antibiotic-resistant bugs that these drugs can no longer fight for us, we need to take our immunity back into our own hands. Protection from infection is a "domestic" (internal immune system) responsibility and should only be "outsourced" (to medicines) rarely and in times of extreme illness.

What to Feed Your Baby for Optimizing Immune Strength

It might be surprising to learn, but 80 percent of our immune system is actually found in the gut. So the best way to keep your baby healthy is by focusing on his gut. Healthy intestines discourage infection. Feed him foods that nourish intestinal tissue, support the mucosal lining (which coats the gut), and provide him plenty of good bacteria in his diet and environment. By building these layers (intestinal tissue, mucosa, good bacteria), you'll be ensuring that he's got a really thick and strong barrier against infecting agents and toxins, so your baby is much less likely to get sick.

The immune system uses nutrients to do its work; therefore, nutrients are critical to staying healthy and avoiding illness. To fight off invaders and infection, the immune system particularly relies on protein; several specific vitamins, minerals and antioxidants; as well as probiotics, the right ratio of good omega fatty acids, and help from antimicrobial fats (for example, those in grass-fed butter, meats, and coconut oil). Without these integral nutrients from whole foods, the immune system is missing critical generals, majors, and lieutenants in the war against outside invaders. Experts warn that *even a single* nutrient deficiency will suppress the immune system, disarming it, and will allow infection to embed more easily. Super Nutrition, rich in Super POWER foods, will cover your baby's immune-nutrient bases.

THE SUNSHINE VITAMIN HELPS IMMUNE PERFORMANCE

Vitamin D is intimately involved with the immune system (see chapter 7). It is found in high concentrations in many kinds of immune cells. According to a study published in the *American Journal of Respiratory and Critical Care Medicine,* a single dose of vitamin D can stop pathogenic bacteria and has been suggested as a treatment for tuberculosis. Vitamin D insufficiency is related to higher rates of common colds, influenza, and the respiratory infection RSV. It likely contributes to the increased rate of illness during darker winter months when we expose our skin to less sunshine.

While sunshine exposure is the best way to acquire sufficient vitamin D, it is also important to get some vitamin D from foods or supplements, especially during the winter months in northern climates. Vitamin D–containing foods include fish roe, fish liver oils, wild-caught fish and shellfish (don't feed to your baby until 18 months), "sun-exposed" animal fats (particularly from chickens and pigs), as well as liver and egg yolks.

POWER UP IMMUNITY WITH PLENTIFUL PROBIOTICS

As previously discussed, good bacteria protects your baby from *bad* bacteria. Too few probiotics means a higher likelihood of infections. According to the textbook *Pediatric Gastroenterology and Clinical Nutrition,* "The primary cause of infection is not due to the presence of unfriendly bacteria, but is actually due to *insufficient* friendly bacteria." [emphasis added]

Good bacteria are *bad* microbes' natural enemy. They fight illness-causing strains of bacteria, yeast, parasites, and *even viruses (like cold and flu).* According to a study in the journal *Pediatrics,* beneficial bacteria are effective in *preventing* childhood colds and flus. Giving probiotics twice a day to 3- to 5-year-olds during 6 months reduced fever incidence by 72 percent!, coughing by 62 percent!, and runny noses by 58 percent! The groups getting probiotics also used fewer antibiotics and missed fewer days of school. Such significant findings imply that *chronic runny noses, coughs, and viral illness in children could actually be caused by a probiotic deficiency.*

Supplemental probiotics are also very helpful for immune and overall health. In *Digestive Wellness: How to Strengthen the Immune System and Prevent Disease through Healthy Digestion,* Elizabeth Lipski, Ph.D., reports on studies that show "supplemental Lactobacillus acidophilus and L. casei decreased the severity and incidence of bronchitis and pneumonia in babies aged six months to two years."

The kind of bacteria your baby is exposed to early on can influence whether or not they will later develop 3Cs, like allergies and asthma. In a 2011 study, reported in the *Journal of Allergy and Clinical Immunology,* lead by John Penders of Maastricht University, 2,700 babies were followed through age seven. Researchers found that a baby's early exposure to bad bacteria (presence of Escherichia coli and Clostridia difficile in their guts) resulted in a higher likelihood that they would have immune-mediated health problems, such as food sensitivities, eczema, and/or wheezing in childhood.

Disinfecting Is Disastrous

Science from two centuries ago taught us to fear all germs. Now, though, we know that germs are mostly *helpful*. Microbes live in our bodies as friendly helpers that act together as another "organ" upon which we rely: without them, we'd die. These friendly flora are defenders and *protect* us from heavy metals, other toxins, and infectious agents; they create nutrients for us and help us digest foods properly.

As noted in the textbook *Pediatric Gastroenterology and Clinical Nutrition*, "There are literally millions of different types of bacteria . . . [only] a very small percentage is actually toxic to humans." Again, most bacteria actually helps your child's immune defenses to be as strong as possible.

Being "sterile" by using disinfectants should not be confused with being "clean." Instead of seeing antibacterial soaps, cleansers, wipes, sprays, and sanitizing gels as ways to protect your baby from "harmful" bugs, view them as products that *kill off* his army of protective microbes, making bad bugs even stronger and your child's defenses even weaker.

Specifically, beware of antibacterial wipes, gels, and soaps with agents like triclosan (aka Microban), a registered pesticide, which accumulates in your child's tissues as other pesticides do. Its use has been linked to higher rates of allergies, immune diseases, organ damage, endocrine malfunction, and eroded immune systems. Kids overexposed to triclosan, for example, have higher rates of hay fever and allergies.

This has led several experts to question these practices, like Dr. Matthew Greenhawt, M.D., Infectious Diseases in Children editorial board member. He ponders, as we do, "in our clean modern-day society, where we protect our children from infection through methods ranging from an aggressive vaccination program to a seemingly omnipresent availability of instant hand sanitizer, one must wonder if our rising rates of allergy and atopic disorders parallel our efforts to *reduce* microbial exposure."

Don't try to make your baby too clean for his own good. By constantly attempting to protect a child from confrontation with bacteria, overprotective parents only serve to reduce the microbial exposure *needed* to cultivate his immune system. And if *some* bad bugs get to him, along with all the good, studies show that mild early-life illness and immune system engagement can create lifelong immunity and ward off autoimmune conditions later in life. *Let him fight his own microbial battles*; he'll be healthier and stronger for it—all his life.

Fun in the Sun

"Uncover Your Baby!" instructs Robert Sears, M.D., in *Happy Baby: The Organic Guide to Baby's First 24 Months*, in order to gain the much-needed vitamin D that is only stimulated by "middle of the day" UV rays, "without sunscreen to block them."

Experts often advise us to slather on the sunblock and minimize our sun exposure during the day's peak hours, but this avoidance of the sun's healthy rays has caused a global vitamin D deficiency, the risks and costs of which far outweigh those of skin cancer (which is often best defended against with a diet rich in antioxidants). Within 15 to 30 minutes in direct sun, a Caucasian baby wearing just a diaper can make 400 IU of vitamin D. Darker-skinned babies need up to five to ten times more time in the sun to make an equivalent amount.

Babies love to be outside in just a diaper and won't get burned in this short amount of time. Rather than toxin-laden drugstore sunscreen, massage coconut oil into his skin, like traditional islanders do. Different from the '80s days of baby oil for "frying" the skin, coconut oil provides your baby mild sun protection while allowing her to get some vitamin D and a tan. (While a tan is helpful sun protection, burning is never okay.)

If you or your baby will be in the sun for extended periods of time, please cover up or use a natural nontoxic sunscreen. Let your baby's skin be kissed by the sun—knowing he's making the vitamin D he needs!

Your baby's intestinal tract is essentially sterile at birth, so the bacteria to which he is exposed early in life have carte blanche to colonize within his gut. You want good bugs to take their rightful place as rulers of his gut ecosystem, establishing a hierarchy that keeps bad bugs at bay. Nature designed the first exposure to be through the vaginal canal, during birth, where a baby is exposed to mom's flora (which doesn't happen if delivery is by Cesarean section). Next, your baby is dosed with even more beneficial bacteria if you nurse because your colustrum and milk are packed with healthy probiotics.

Early exposure to such healthy bacteria serves him well by protecting against infection (as well as facilitating digestion, getting rid of toxins, making vitamins, and more!). Also, as Penders' study showed, babies with healthy bacteria (known to actively crowd out bad bacteria) are not as likely to have allergies and asthma in childhood, as are those babies born via C-section who have pathogenic bacteria taking up residence in their intestinal tract. If your baby had a C-section delivery or is not being nursed, it is critical to supplement directly with probiotics and to include lacto-fermented foods and raw and cultured dairy early on in his

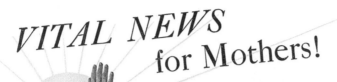

VITAL NEWS
for Mothers!

Bond Bread
now brings
sunshine vitamin-D

*Never before supplied in sufficient quantity
by any table-food—now this scarcest
of health-guarding elements can
be had at every meal.*

If your child went naked in the noon-day sun, any kind of bread might do.

TO BUILD strong bones and sound even teeth, to promote proper growth, to strengthen resistance to colds and illness, everybody — especially children —needs sunshine vitamin-D every day. But until now enough of it could be obtained only from direct sunshine, from sun-lamps, and from medicines.

Now scientists have found a way to provide this vital, health-building food element in bread. And Bond Bread has been chosen exclusively to offer you the benefits of this discovery. They guarantee that one to two slices of Bond Bread at each meal will give you all the extra sunshine vitamin-D you need.

Ask your grocer for sunshine vitamin-D Bond Bread—the same home-like flavor, the same firm texture that Flavor-Peak

Rising insures—the bread that more than a million housewives buy every day. And with this priceless improvement, it costs you no more than you have been paying.

**OFFICIALLY APPROVED BY
HIGHEST AUTHORITIES**

Every claim made in this advertisement has been specifically checked and approved by recognized scientific authority. Bond Bread, analyzed and tested as to its sunshine vitamin-D content, has been granted the official seals of acceptance and approval of the following:

THE AMERICAN MEDICAL ASSO-
CIATION'S COMMITTEE ON FOODS
Wisconsin Alumni Research Foundation
Good Housekeeping Bureau of Foods
Physical Culture Institute
Home-Making Center
The Paediatrics Research Foundation
Child Health Magazine
Parents' Magazine
Guaranteed by
The General Baking Company

Write to General Baking Company, Suite 962, 420 Lexington Avenue, New York City for this booklet.

The Sunshine Trail to HAPPIER HEALTH

Bond Bread *

© 1931, G. B. Co.

FOR HAPPIER HEALTH look for the above emblem that marks each Bond Bread wrapper . . . Bond Bread and Bond Bakers Whole Wheat are the *only* breads that give you the extra sunshine vitamin-D you need . . .

December 1931 Good Housekeeping

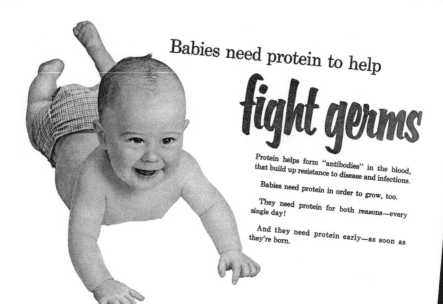

Babies need protein to help

fight germs

Protein helps form "antibodies" in the blood, that build up resistance to disease and infections.

Babies need protein in order to grow, too.

They need protein for both reasons—every single day!

And they need protein early—as soon as they're born.

There's plenty of protein in these **meats!**

There's 5 times more protein than the usual babies' meat "soups," and 10 times more than even mother's milk, ounce for ounce!

And Swift's Meats for Babies are pre-cooked and strained so fine babies can eat them when they're just 3 weeks old.

A recent clinical study indicated meat-fed babies had fewer colds.

Help your baby fight germs from the inside. Give him more protein. Get Swift's Meats today.

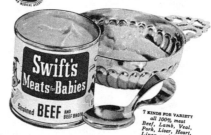

7 KINDS FOR VARIETY
all 100% meat
Beef, Lamb, Veal,
Pork, Liver, Heart,
Liver-and-Bacon

Swift's Meats for Babies

 New! Ready to serve egg yolks for baby! No more daily egg cooking for baby! Here's Swift's Strained Egg Yolks for Babies, already cooked and ready to serve, right out of the can. Give baby needed iron this new convenient way.

92

diet to ensure adequate exposure and colonization of beneficial bacteria. (Note: also avoid using antibacterial agents.)

Lacto-fermented foods and beverages, fresh (raw) dairy, and cultured dairy (e.g., yogurt and kefir) are sources of probiotics as well as lactic acid, which is very helpful for intestinal (and therefore immune) health. Traditional cultures benefited from extra probiotics in foods long before contemporary medicine "discovered" them. Before refrigeration, foods were preserved through lacto-fermentation, which not only kept spoilage at bay but offered the very real benefits of being rich in *probiotics*, *antioxidants*, *enzymes*, and *lactic acid*. Eating these foods regularly helped with digestion and strengthened the immune system, keeping these traditional children more robust and healthier than the chronically sick children we see too often today.

The flora that your baby has introduced to his gut now will determine his long-term immune capabilities. In the first two years of life, varied microbial exposure and probiotic-rich foods will influence a lifetime of health. By using the recipes we recommend in this and other chapters, you'll naturally support optimal development of your baby's immune system and strength against pathogens.

ENABLE ENZYMES TO ENGAGE THE ENEMY

Strive to supply your baby with enzyme-rich foods as a great way to fortify his immunity. Enzymes support white blood cells and other infection-fighting agents, while directly fighting pathogens, too. Fortunately, many

of the probiotic-rich foods are also enzyme-rich foods. Fresh, raw milk is an excellent source of enzyme-based pathogen killers. Tropical fruits, like pineapple, kiwi, and papaya, and lacto-fermented foods and beverages, like sauerkraut and cultured dairy (yogurt), provide enzymes as well.

A WELL-ROUNDED TRADITIONAL-FOODS DIET STRENGTHENS IMMUNE FUNCTION

By feeding your baby plenty of good fats—particularly saturated fats—you'll provide him with antiviral, antibacterial, and antimicrobial fatty acids that will help him stay healthy. The Weston A. Price Foundation reports that butter contains glycosphingolipids, which specifically protect against intestinal infection, especially in the very young. Butter fats, as well as the fats in coconut oil, have antimicrobial constituents that are active against pathogens and yeast, while feeding good bacteria.

Protein- and nutrient-rich foods are broken down into amino acids, which your baby's body will use to build his immune army (antibodies). There is a reason chicken soup is seen as a panacea of healing—not just for the soul, but for the body as well. The protein, fats, highly absorbable minerals, and gelatin in soup (made with bones) are restorative and supportive to the digestive system and thus critical to immunity. Protein deficiency stunts the body's ability to build enzymes and antibodies, both of which are necessary for immune function and fighting off illness.

What *Not* to Feed Your Baby for Optimizing Immune Strength

Avoiding flour- and sugar-based foods and other inflammation-causing foods will increase the chances that your baby's immune potential will be reached.

SUGAR: NOT SO SWEET FOR PROTECTION FROM INFECTION

Sugar, particularly, increases the body's susceptibility to infection. Jerry Kartzinel, M.D., pediatrician and coauthor of *Healing and Preventing Autism*, states, "the best way to get . . . [the] immune system to improve is to DECREASE . . . SUGAR INTAKE!" [emphasis *not* added] As published in the *Journal of Clinical Nutrition*, sugar—including honey, juice, glucose, sucrose (table sugar), and fructose (in juice, high fructose corn syrup, and fruit) all *significantly* reduce your baby's immune system's ability to destroy pathogenic bacteria.

Sugar and white flour are the favorite foods of many bad bugs and yeasts. These pathogenic flora feed on such simple carbs and ferment them in the gut, causing gas, diarrhea, and intestinal illness. By eliminating refined carbohydrates in your baby's diet, you reduce these sickness-causing flora by starving them.

FOODS THAT FEED THE FIRES OF INFLAMMATION

Foods that cause inflammation weaken your baby's immune system, making it hard for good flora to make a home. Inflammation is affected by the ratio of essential fatty acids you get in your diet. Omega-3 fatty acids directly reduce inflammation and thin the blood in the body, whereas most omega-6 fatty acids cause inflammation and platelet stickiness. While both are integral to health, it is the *ratio* of omega-3 to omega-6 fatty acids, as well as the "nutritiousness" of the fat they come in, that is most important.

Russel L. Blaylock, M.D., reports on studies showing that inflammatory-inducing omega-6 fats reduce immune capabilities. He notes, "We now know that omega-6 oils profoundly suppress immunity . . . as a result they also promote infections."

In our modern diet, there are far too many unhealthy omega-6s (found in vegetable oils and grain-fed animal foods) and far too few omega-3s (fish oils, flaxseed oil, grass-fed/pastured animal foods), resulting in an inflammatory imbalance. (Most Americans get twenty to fifty omega-6s for every one omega-3.) A traditional-foods diet, however, will naturally provide the correct omega-fatty-acid ratio.

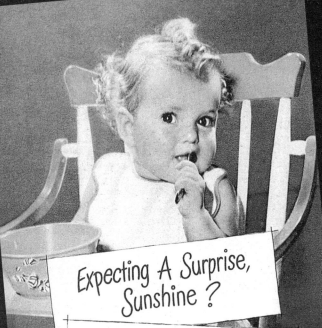

Expecting A Surprise, Sunshine ?

OKAY! HERE IT COMES—DOUBLE GOOD, TOO! Custard all tastily "trimmed" with Strained Peaches (*both*, Gerber's). There's no end of happy mealtime surprises for baby—when mommy and *Gerber's wider-than-ever variety* get together.

JUST WHAT THE DOCTOR ORDERED— VARIETY! More and more, doctors say "Baby likes variety." And, baby needs a variety of minerals and vitamins— even from her first solid food after milk (usually Cereal). That's why all Gerber's, Cereals, Fruits, Vegetables and Desserts are specially prepared to retain precious nutrients—*and* the palatable flavor babies go for.

"GOOD THINGS COME IN SMALL PACKAGES!"— like Gerber's Junior Foods. Same size container, same low price as Gerber's Strained. So, baby gets more variety—you have fewer leftovers, lower grocery bills—with good-tasting Gerber's!

Free! Samples of Gerber's 3 Cereals. Write to Dept. 15-8, Gerber's, Fremont, Mich.

Babies are our business... our only business!

Gerber's
BABY FOODS
Fremont, Mich. — Oakland, Cal.

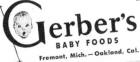

3 CEREALS • 20 STRAINED FOODS • 15 JUNIOR FOODS

88

If Your Baby Does Get Sick

The reason humans have an immune system is to fight infection, and it is inevitable that sometimes your baby *will* get sick—and *should*, on occasion. Typically fed babies are reported to catch seven to ten colds per year, which is more frequent than one would expect in a traditionally nourished baby. Providing Super Nutrition should improve your baby's immune capability and minimize infection frequency, as well as severity. When your baby does get sick, honor his instincts to eat (or not), but ensure that he drinks and stays hydrated.

CHOOSE BEVERAGES WISELY

Diarrhea can drain the body of minerals, such as potassium and sodium—which is why your pediatrician often recommends commercial electrolyte solutions. These beverages, however, are bad enough for *well* children, but are even worse for sick kids because they contain immune-hampering sugar, high fructose corn syrup, and artificial dyes and sweeteners with very little "real" nutrition.

Coconut water, however, is a natural source of nutrient-rich hydration and is an excellent way to replace lost electrolytes during illness. Coconut water has even been used successfully as a direct IV fluid in wartime during supply shortages. Another premier electrolyte solution is Souper Stock (page 56). We recommend alternating coconut water (see page 93) with Souper Stock during illness. (For younger babies, mom's milk is the very best fluid during illness, with homemade formula being second best. See page 204.) Coconut water or mom's milk can also be frozen into ice pops to soothe sore throats and provide hydration.

STARVE A FEVER

The old adage "starve a fever, feed a cold" has some scientific credence. Studies show that babies instinctually do not choose to eat when they have a fever. A 36–48 hour fast can actually result in a significant boost to the immune system's infection-fighting capabilities. Temporarily not feeling hungry and therefore not eating much while sick might allow his immune system to function better. Although we don't ever suggest that you make your baby fast, we offer this information to help reassure you that if your child is not eating for a day or two, as long as he is drinking, you need not be over-worried.

During such time, offer him fats, such as marrow, ghee, butter, or tiny spoonfuls of coconut oil. Fats such as these are rich in natural antimicrobial, antiviral, and antibacterial agents, and just small amounts can be satiating, preventing hunger pangs. Also, a fat-rich diet lessens dehydration risk.

Trust the Wisdom of the Baby Body

In the 1920s and '30s, pediatrician Clara Davis, M.D., did a six-year feeding experiment with babies beginning at age 6 to 11 months. In September 1939, she published her results, entitled "The Self-Selection of Diets by Young Children," in the *Canadian Medical Association Journal*.

She provided the babies and children with nutrient-dense, real foods, including soured milk, sea salt, bananas, orange juice, barley, cornmeal, peaches, bone jelly (gelatinous bone-stock), tomatoes, beets, meats, bone marrow, raw lettuce, cooked and raw eggs, oatmeal, wheat, peas, cabbage, apples, and cooked glandular organs, lamb, and chicken. Babies were allowed to choose as much of whatever was before them.

Though their individual choices varied widely and changed over time, all the babies were hale, hearty, and "throve." None were noticeably fat or thin. There were no constipation issues, no vomiting, no diarrhea, and no serious illness, though once the group did get a fever. (Interestingly, during this illness, most chose unusually high amounts of *raw* beef, carrots, and beets.)

None of the babies developed nutrient-deficiency diseases. In fact, some who'd entered the study with rickets (a vitamin D-related mineral deficiency disease) cured themselves of it by choosing foods that were rich in vitamin D. Interestingly, when their rickets was cured, they stopped focusing on these foods.

The babies self-selected foods in the right quantities and variety to ensure they had all essential nutrients, adequate energy, and proper digestive health. Dr. Davis called this "the wisdom of the body," though she warned, "self-selection can have no ... value if the diet ... [is] selected from inferior foods" like white flour and sugar and their "train of nutritional evils."

In fact, all fifteen babies in the study were superbly healthy. Dr. Davis quotes another doctor (for purposes of unbiased reporting) on the state of health of the children in her study, as published in the *Journal of Pediatrics*: "They were the finest group of specimens from the physical and behavior standpoint that I have ever seen in children at that age."

Your baby, too, has "wisdom" of his body—and you *can* trust it. He wants to eat foods that will uniquely meet the needs of *his* growing body and mind. He can do this, but only if you provide him with nourishing PURE and Super POWER foods.

REBALANCE GUT ECOSYSTEM AFTER ANTIBIOTICS TO AVOID REPEAT INFECTIONS

Antibiotics damage the immune system by killing good bacteria and creating the right environment for bad microbes to thrive. This leaves your baby's immune system in a weakened state, more susceptible to repeat infections, and allows for overgrowth of antibiotic-resistant bacteria and other microbes, like yeast. After antibiotics, it is very important to rebuild healthy flora and regain a favorable balance in the intestinal ecosystem by providing your baby's body with probiotic-rich foods and supplements (see page 96). When antibiotics are necessary, be sure to supplement with probiotics, according to package directions, and incorporate lacto-fermented foods and beverages (see chapter 2) daily, for at least one month after antibiotic treatment.

Stave Off Infection by Steering Clear of Baby Food Jars and Pasta Pitfalls

Part of your baby's burgeoning independence is learning more about himself, his personality, his likes and dislikes—including foods and things related to feeding. Provide a variety of real foods on his high chair tray and let him self-select the foods that will best nourish him at that meal or on that day.

If you *only* provide your baby with meals of nutrient-rich, real, whole foods, you need not stress about quantity and variety; your baby will eat when he is hungry and needs nutrients. If, however, his diet includes sugar, white flour, or juice, you cannot rely on his hunger cues and preferences since these foods can be addictive and make him feel full without actually providing enough nutrition.

We, along with the AAP, recommend offering *many* different foods by the end of the first year, as there is nutritional value in variety. Yet the typical diet at this age is limited, including mainly stage 3 jarred foods and grain-based foods, like O-shaped cereal, crackers, and pasta. According to the AAP, if you don't offer many different foods, then you will be limiting "important sources of nutrients . . . and could compromise nutritional status."

Additionally, variety in the diet helps broaden children's palates and helps to instill positive eating habits early. Offer a new food eight to thirty times before giving up, as it takes time for babies to become familiar with new tastes and textures.

We recommend significantly limiting (or avoiding altogether) refined salt and sugar for babies this age. Refined salt, like table salt and the kind you find in packaged foods, is simply sodium chloride. This kind of salt is very disturbing to the body because most of the naturally occurring minerals found in whole salt are stripped away during refining and processing. Beware: Even baby-and "kid-foods" can include harmful flavor boosters in them.

Pattern	10 Months
Early AM	Mom's milk /homemade formula, then meal (shortly after waking)
Mid-Morning	Milk / homemade formula
Mid-Day	Meal
Afternoon	Milk / homemade formula (before nap)
Evening	Meal
Nighttime	Milk / homemade formula (before bed)

Pattern	11 Months
Early AM	Mom's milk /homemade formula, then meal (shortly after waking
Mid-Morning	Snack
Mid-Day	Meal
Afternoon	Milk / homemade formula (before nap)
Evening	Meal
Nighttime	Milk / homemade formula (before bed)

Unrefined salt, however, is good for your baby (and for you!). Adding a pinch of high-quality sea salt to water makes it an electrolyte solution, and adding sea salt to Souper Stock (page 56) means it is rich in both *macro*minerals from bones and *micro*minerals from the salt. Whole salt is actually essential for life and good for health. This kind of salt is made of *eighty* highly absorbable trace minerals that occur naturally in proportions that make them work best together and in the body (so the health problems often seen with refined salt are not seen with sea salt). Particularly, unrefined salt is important for proper digestion and nutrient assimilation and thus serves to bolster the immune system. Celtic sea salt or Himalayan salt are our preferred brand, being richest in mineral content. Redmond Real Salt is also mineral rich. Whole salt should have color—usually beige, gray, or pink—whereas "table" salt is white due to processing, refining, and bleaching.

PRACTICAL FEEDING TIPS AT THIS AGE

Faster introduction, thicker consistency. New foods can now be given every one or two days, rather than every three or four. Also, foods can now be of a much more "chunky" consistency and need not be thinned down. Though many commercial baby foods are "microwavable," we absolutely do *not* recommend heating your baby's food in the microwave.

Super Nutrition Food Categorizations for 10 to 12 Months

Super POWER	PURE
Lacto-fermented fruits and veggies	Organic tropical fruits
Coconut kefir	Coconut water, unsweetened
Grass-fed, raw cheese	Onion, garlic, beets, and other organic fruits and
Kidneys and other organ meats	vegetables
Cod liver oil	Organic meats, eggs, and other animal foods
Animal fats from grass-fed animals	

OKAY	CRAP
Organic baby food (stage 3)	Pretzels, crackers, cookies, bars
Nonorganic, non–Dirty Dozen fruits and vegetables, washed	Prepared baby "meals"
All-natural meats, eggs, and other animal foods	Noodles and pasta dishes
Nonpastured, nonorganic animal fats	Sweetened baby foods
	Juice
	Pasteurized dairy

Even though you need not be as concerned with straining, puréeing, and thinning, your baby still isn't ready to handle chewing and swallowing like a grown-up. Choking is a risk, so never leave your child unattended while eating.

Family meals. Around this age, your baby's meals will align with family mealtimes, as he will be eating three times per day now. Though it's often easiest to feed your baby first, and then eat, we advise that you eat with your baby starting from an early age. A bite for baby, then a bite for you—if possible. Despite the mess, keep offering your baby a spoon. The added weight and thicker texture of these new foods now may make it easier for your baby to find success when using it!

Water. Hydration is tantamount to proper bodily function and detoxification. Offer filtered water in between meals. However, refrain from offering too much at meals. Too much water can reduce stomach acid, which is necessary for proper protein digestion. Souper Stock, mom's milk, cultured mommy milk, or formula can be offered in a cup through the day or with meals.

Foods and fluids. Babies normally take between 18 and 24 ounces (520 to 710 ml) of mom's milk or formula at this age, meeting approximately one-third to one-half of their caloric needs.

If your baby consistently doesn't want to eat much, he may be drinking too much mom's milk or homemade/enriched formula. While these are the most nourishing beverages available and are still a critical part of his diet, his growing nutrient needs mandate that he *also* eat nutritious foods.

Experts advise that babies should not drink pasteurized cow's milk at this age, and we agree due to its increased risk of anemia, iron deficiency, gastrointestinal bleeding, and allergies and intolerance. Fresh, raw, unpasteurized milk, however, from a trusted grass-fed source does not carry such risks. Even with this high-caliber dairy, we still feel one year is the appropriate age to offer cow's milk to drink, unless it is part of a recipe for homemade formula (as recommended in chapter 8).

Fluctuating appetite. Be aware that your baby's appetite can fluctuate, and his likes and dislikes can change. If he's not eating much, choose foods that pack the most-nutrient-dense punch in the smallest quantity, namely Super POWER foods; organ meats, fish eggs, grass-fed raw butter, and raw yogurt are all foods that provide superb nutrition and plenty of energy—even if only a few bites make their way into his tummy.

Mom to Mom / When your baby begins eating more than one food at a meal, we advise including animal protein or at least an animal fat at each meal. Avoid making meals out of only fruits, or only fruits and vegetables. Side dishes should be vegetables ideally three times a day (i.e., one with each meal), and fruits no more than twice a day (e.g., snack and dessert).

Recipes to Optimize Immunity

Popular snack foods like cereal and crackers are typically introduced at this age. Introducing these foods will often make them instant "favorites," with babies preferring them over more nutritious options. Even if your baby can't yet talk, he may communicate his desire for such foods through tantrums and crying. These products usually don't offer many nutrients, they aren't worth eating, and you'd be better off allowing your child to become hungry enough (within reason) to accept more nutritious offerings.

Between 10 and 12 months, you can introduce beets, cooked berries, fish, coconut water, and raw cheese. For a more complete list of acceptable foods at this age, see the Food Introduction Timeline on page 222.

Mashed Not-Potatoes

Since white potatoes are part of the nightshade family—which can cause inflammation—we don't recommend them yet. Either taro (a tuber) or cauliflower can be used to make a mashed potato–like side dish without the "risk." Part of Polynesian cuisine, taro must be well cooked.

Mashed Cauliflower:

1 crown cauliflower

Butter or ghee to taste

Celtic sea salt to taste

Steam the cauliflower until mushy.
Drain the water.
Purée with the butter or ghee and sea salt until desired consistency.

Yield: About 1 cup (225 g)

Mashed Taro:

2 to 4 taro roots

Ghee, butter, or other Fabulous Fat (see page 176) to taste

Celtic sea salt to taste

Preheat the oven to 300°F (150°C, gas mark 2).
Bake the taro for 1 hour. When cool enough to handle, peel. Mash with fat of choice and sea salt.

Optional: Add coconut milk or grated hard, raw cheese (such as Colby or cheddar).

Yield: About 1 cup (225 g)

Mashed Poi (Fermented Taro Root):

2 teaspoons whey, OR ¼ cup (60 ml) water + ½ packet (¼ tablespoon) of culture starter + ½ teaspoon Rapunzel brand Rapadura* or other whole-foods sweetener that has sat for 20 minutes

1 cup (225 g) baked, peeled, mashed taro from previous recipe

Mix ingredients in glass bowl and place in a mason jar on a counter, sealed, for 24 hours. Serve as a side dish to meat.

Yield: About 1 cup (225 g)

Notes
- Taro can replace potato in many recipes.
- *Rapadura is a mineral-containing sugar, found at health food stores or online.

Fromage Frais (Fresh, Unpasteurized Cheese)

Cheese is a complete food that alone can sustain life. We prefer raw cheese over pasteurized cheese. In fact, we hesitate to recommend pasteurized dairy in any form until the age of 2, with the exception of yogurt or kefir when raw dairy is not available.

Raw cheese can be found at your local health food store or from a trusted, grass-fed raw dairy source. Raw dairy is packed with minerals and sustains enzymes that would otherwise be lost during pasteurization—both of these nutritional factors make fresh, raw cheese an excellent dietary constituent for immune support.

"Offal"-Good Kidneys

Offal comes from the words "off fall," as in the parts of the animal that "fall off" during preparation and butchering. Offal is a catchall term for what we typically call organ meats, such as kidneys, liver, tripe, giblets, and various other organs. Kidneys are nearly as nutritious as liver. If they were to make it back to the modern dinner table, the nutrition they offer would protect children from toxins and nutrient-deficiency complications, including many of the 3C conditions we see today.

Nutrition abounds in offal, particularly liver and kidneys. (Kidneys have more vitamin C than pears or apples!) Choose offal from organic, grass-fed animals on a pastured farm (see Resources, page 218). Organ meats are more nutrient dense, by far, than muscle meats. Nutrients are absolutely essential to optimal immune function, and regularly incorporating organ meats in your baby's diet will support strong immunity and also optimal growth and development of other systems.

1 finely diced onion

2 tablespoons (28 g) butter

2 kidneys (chicken, beef, or pork), thinly sliced

¹/₂ cup (120 ml) Souper Stock (page 56)

In a sauté pan over medium heat, cook the onions in the butter until very soft and brown. Add the kidneys and heat through. Add the Souper Stock and heat through.

Remove from heat and add to blender or food processor. Purée, adding more stock, if necessary, for the correct consistency.

Yield: 2 to 4 servings, depending on size of kidneys

Sweet Potato Pancakes or "Crackers"

These sweet potato treats can be made into either pancakes or crackers. The vibrant orange hue in sweet potatoes hints at the great array of antioxidants contained within, which will support overall health and wellness in many ways. Nutmeg is not part of the nut family and is not allergenic, as tree nuts are.

For Pancakes:

4 tablespoons (55 g) butter, ghee, or coconut oil

1 egg yolk

Pinch nutmeg

¹/₄ cup (55 g) previously baked sweet potato (see page 62)

¹/₈ teaspoon Celtic sea salt

2 tablespoons (28 g) butter, ghee, or coconut oil

¹/₄ cup (28 g) (heaping) coconut flour (or unsweetened, unsulfured, finely shredded coconut)

Warm the 4 tablespoons (55 g) fat in a cast-iron skillet. In a bowl, mix the egg yolk, nutmeg, sweet potato, salt, 2 tablespoons (28 g) fat, and coconut flour.

Roll the mixture into 1- to 1¹/₂-inch (2.5 × 3.8 cm) balls and flatten between your palms before placing into the hot pan.

Cook and flip the "cakes" a few times on each side, flattening with a spatula. Cook until browned and heated through, about 10 to 12 minutes.

Yield: 4 to 6 pancakes

For Crackers:

1 egg yolk

Pinch nutmeg

½ cup (115 g) previously baked sweet potato (see page 62)

2 teaspoons water

¼ cup (28 g) coconut flour (or unsweetened, unsulfured, finely shredded coconut)

Ghee or butter

Preheat the oven to 325°F (170°C, gas mark 3).

In a bowl, mix the egg yolk, nutmeg, sweet potato, water, and coconut flour.

Grease a stainless steel cookie sheet with ghee or butter (or use greased parchment paper if using an aluminum cookie sheet). Using wet hands, flatten the dough into a thin (⅛ inch or 0.3 cm) rectangle and place on the cookie sheet.

Bake for 15 to 20 minutes and then flip and bake on other side for 15 to 20 minutes more.

Let cool and then cut or break into bite-size crackers for baby.

Yield: About 12 crackers

Notes
- The crackers make a great on-the-go snack.
- Particularly delicious are the crackers warm, spread with raw butter!

Coconut Water/Coconut Kefir

Coconut water, the "sap" within the coconut that has not yet turned into coconut meat (copra), is rich in nutrients and minerals. It is an excellent occasional beverage for your baby. Young coconut water has the same electrolyte (mineral) balance as human blood and thus is a natural hydrating "sports" drink as well as an immune-supporting beverage. It also has potassium that works to keep a healthy blood pressure level. Purchase unsweetened coconut water at your health food store or online at Body Ecology (see Resources, page 218). (For a fun project, you can "make" coconut water by cracking a whole, young, green coconut.)

By culturing coconut water into coconut kefir, even more immune benefits are conferred, including lactic acid, more probiotics, and even enzymes! Add a kefir starter packet (see Resources, page 218) to coconut water and allow fermentation to occur at room temperature (following the kefir packet directions). Also, you can purchase coconut kombucha (see chapter 7) from your health food store or coco-biotic fermented coconut water drink from Body Ecology.

Berry-Scrumptious Berries

In a few months, you can introduce raw berries, but until then, they must still be cooked to ensure your baby has a chance to digest them. Start with strawberries and blueberries at this age. Add blackberries, raspberries, marionberries, juneberries, and fresh mulberries around

15 months of age. Serving berries with plain (preferably raw) yogurt makes a nice, digestible parfait, or you can make Finger-Fun Gelatin Jigglers (page 85). Dark purple berries are rich in resveratrol, a powerful antioxidant, anti-carcinogenic, and anti-inflammatory compound, which supports the immune system. Cook 1 cup (145 g) fresh or frozen berries in a small saucepan over medium-low heat until the berries until soft. Stir occasionally and mash the fruit or purée off heat.

Beet Soup

Beets are known as builders and cleansers of the blood. Betacyanin (an antioxidant) is the phytonutrient that gives beets their deep amethyst hue. One of the foods babies chose when sick in Clara Davis's studies (see page 105), beets are rich in nutrients that support the immune system. This recipe is adapted from Nourishing Traditions *by Sally Fallon.*

2 tablespoons (28 g) butter, marrow, ghee, coconut oil, or (26 g) lard

1 tablespoon (3 g) chopped chives

3 beets, peeled and finely chopped

1 garlic clove, minced

1 stalk celery, minced, optional

1/2 quart (475 ml) filtered water

Warm the fat in a large pot over medium heat.

Add the chives, beets, garlic, and celery, if using. Sauté until soft, about 30 minutes.

Add the water and simmer for 15 to 20 minutes until the vegetables are soft. Remove from heat. Purée with an immersion blender or put in a blender. (Take caution when blending hot liquids.)

Yield: 3 adult servings, or two mom-and-baby servings

Notes
- This soup can be very messy. It's best to feed this to a shirtless baby!
- It's very important to purchase organic beets, as nonorganic beets are high in nitrates.

Schmaltz and Gribenes

Rendered chicken fat is called "schmaltz" in traditional Jewish cooking. Gribenes are a bonus "by-product" of schmaltz making (as are "crispins" in lard rendering). You can sauté chicken liver with schmaltz and gribenes to round out the nutritional value of the dish. Animal fats, such as schmaltz, offer a buffet of important fatty acids that are immune supporting. This recipe is adapted from The Shiksa in the Kitchen, *online.*

For Schmaltz:

1 pound (455 g) chicken with all skin and fat

Rinse the chicken and chop into 1/2-inch (1 cm) pieces. Fry the pieces over low heat for 15 minutes.

Remove the pan from the heat and drain the liquid fat through a mesh strainer, reserving the strainer contents. The golden oil is the schmaltz.

For Gribenes:

1 large onion, chopped

Celtic sea salt and pepper to taste

After straining the oil, add the onion and put the remaining meat and chicken skin back into the frying pan. Season with sea salt and pepper.

Sauté for about 20 minutes (pieces will darken, but should not blacken).

Yield: 1 cup (235 ml) schmaltz; 2 cups (280 g) gribenes

Notes

- Schmaltz is liquid at room temperature and solid when cold. Use it to sauté foods like liver, added to liver to make chopped liver, or eat just with gribenes.
- Use gribenes as a topping for salads or other dishes (for you), or serve as a great snack for your baby.

Pretty Pink Drink (Beet Kvass)

Beets are very nutrient rich, and many experts say that consuming a bit of beets daily will provide an influx of nutrition and provide support for detoxification and digestion since they have special constituents that support clean blood and the flow of bile from the gallbladder. Beet kvass is a common traditional Ukrainian beverage, also used in vinaigrettes and in soups. It is a health tonic, superb for supporting digestion. This recipe is adapted from Nourishing Traditions *by Sally Fallon and is a Super POWER food.*

1 large organic beet, peeled and finely chopped

1½ tablespoons (25 ml) whey (see Homemade Whey, page 64)

1 teaspoon Celtic sea salt

Place the ingredients in a mason jar. Tamp down.

Add filtered water to nearly fill a 1-quart (950 ml) mason jar and stir well.

Leave sealed on the counter for 2 days and then store in the refrigerator.

Yield: 1 quart (950 ml)

Note

- This can be a beverage option for your baby in small quantities at this age. It is much preferred over juice of any kind.

Shape Up Sweets and Ship Out Sugar

Getting Back to Nature's Basics

12 to 18 Months

Happy birthday to your baby! So much has happened during this first year. Your feeding practices have set a solid foundation for your baby's life-long health—congratulations! But don't hang up the apron just yet; your work is far from over.

Remember that your baby's digestive system is still not comparable to that of a grown-up. She should still be eating a special diet rather than just smaller portions of what you might be having for dinner. (Though you can certainly serve your family larger portions of what you are feeding *her* for dinner.) At 12 months, 50 percent of her calories should still come from mom's milk or formula, with an average intake of 20 to 24 ounces (570 to 710 ml) of formula per day or with nursing at least four times per 24 hours. As you increase her solid food intake, limit—or preferably, omit—refined and processed sugars. If you don't, you're setting her up for developing 3C conditions, most notably diabetes and obesity.

At 12 months, many babies are indoctrinated into the world of adulterated foods, with sugar, white flour, trans fats, refined salt, colors, dyes, and flavorings part of everyday meals and snacks. In this chapter, we'll try to keep you on the traditional-foods path, with ways of feeding your one-year-old with more pure, whole foods, relying on Nature's basics to supply her with a nourishing diet.

Beware of Sugar

Kids and candy seem to go together like peanut butter and jelly. Despite its happy associations, sugar is not as harmless as you might believe. Rather than being a treat or distraction, medical and scientific research supports that sugar is *devastating* to health. Yet sugar intake has been drastically increasing over the last centuries and—notably—has escalated even more in just the last few decades. Kids eat more sugar today than any generation of children before them.

Few parents realize that the FDA, the U.S. Department of Agriculture's Dietary Guidelines, the World Health Organization, and the American Heart Association (AHA) all formally recommend that, in order to be healthy, people limit the amount of added sugars they consume in a day. If sugar were harmless, this wouldn't be necessary. For example, the AHA advises that women should consume no more than 6 teaspoons (about 30 grams or 100 calories) of added sugar per day—which is less than one can of soda pop! Though no specific recommendations are made for children, cutting the adult limits in half for them makes sense.

In terms of Super Nutrition's foundational pillars, processed and sugar-filled foods are the *antithesis* of traditional foods: Sugar hinders digestion, is so far from "pure" it's toxic, impairs immunity, and is the opposite of "nutrient worthy."

SUGAR HURTS DIGESTION

Sugar is scientifically proven to alter mineral balances. Imbalanced minerals are unable to function properly, as they rely on each other in specific proportions. Because minerals are helpers to enzymes, when minerals are imbalanced, enzymes don't function appropriately as they should, and when enzymes can't do their job, then digestion is significantly affected. When foods aren't digested, food allergies are likely to develop, which is why foods that are eaten with sugar are more likely to have allergies developed against them.

SUGAR IS A DRUG AND A TOXIN

It's hard to imagine cupcakes and apple juice being as toxic to the liver as alcohol, as well as a significant contributor to our most dreaded diseases. Yet, while sugar offers energy in the form of calories, it provides nothing to help us grow, heal, or support our body; it changes bodily functions; and its prolonged absence causes withdrawal symptoms. By definition, sugar is much closer to *a drug* than it is to food.

Sugar's effects are similar to those of drugs. Here's a top ten list on how and why:

10. Sugar gives pleasure differently than food; we celebrate and commemorate with it (like alcohol), and we like to "push" it on others (*go on . . . just have one bite!*).
9. Sugar is addicting (we can become "sugarholics").
8. Going without sugar causes withdrawal, both emotional and physical, symptoms, such as irritability, headache, tremors, and moodiness.

7. Sugar affects mood and behavior (disappointed without dessert, having a candy bar after a hard day at work, parents saying their kids are "high on sugar").

6. Ingesting sugar creates an emotional response (joy, relief, pleasure, feeling "better" or less "down").

5. Sugar alters normal endocrine, metabolic, neurologic, and biochemical functioning.

4. Sugar consumption is often hidden from others (e.g., empty ice cream containers buried at the bottom of the garbage, candy bars stashed in sock drawers).

3. Sugar use causes feelings of guilt and embarrassment.

2. Cravings arise when going without sugar for too long.

But the #1 similarity between sugar and drugs is that it stimulates the body via the same mechanisms. Sugar works on the very same neurotransmitters (or brain communicators) that antidepressants, morphine, cocaine/crack, and stimulants affect.

▸ Prozac, Cymbalta . . . and SUGAR affect serotonin.
▸ Morphine, opium, heroin . . . and SUGAR cause an opioid response.
▸ Crack, cocaine . . . and SUGAR cause their high by affecting dopamine.
▸ Caffeine, methamphetamines . . . and SUGAR trigger adrenaline and norepinephrine release.

Sugar is not love, and the "happy" feelings it elicits are only the "high" it induces due to effects on neurotransmitters. When you give in and give your child sweets, you are analagous to a dealer giving a fix.

For such a harmful dietary component, it is a shame that our children's intake is going up and up. Part of the more recent jump in sugar intake is related to the creation of high fructose corn syrup in the 1970s. Over the last 10 decades, as Robert Lustig, M.D., a pediatric neuroendocrinologist and professor, reports, daily fructose consumption has gone from 15 grams to 75 grams (that's like going from having one can of soda pop per day to having five!). Your baby might not be drinking soda pop, but there are 26 grams (over 2 tablespoons!) of sugar in her 7-ounce (200 ml) *juice box*.

When you consider *no* dietary sugar is esssential, any sugar your child consumes is unecessary. If you think "moderation" is still okay, you might want to reconsider your definition of moderation. Counting *all* sugars, including white flour, juice, and others (see sidebar on page 119), it's clear that "sugars" are not only *present* at every meal and snack but actually compose *the majority* of children's diets today. The reality is that just one 2-ounce (55 g) kid-friendly yogurt tube has more than 2 teaspoons of sugar (10 grams), a serving of typical breakfast cereal has 3 teaspoons of sugar (15 grams), and 1 pouch of fruit-flavored snacks has over 3 teaspoons of sugar (15 grams). Unless you make a serious effort to control and reduce sugars, your child will consume *far in excess* of moderation just eating normal "kid" foods.

Both sugar (sucrose) and high fructose corn syrup are double sugars made of both glucose and fructose. The damage of too much glucose has been studied and reported, including metabolic syndrome and risk of heart disease, diabetes, and obesity—all of which are related to the insulin response triggered by excess glucose.

As this 1952 ad says, "Hey, take it easy, Junior! Here comes a big dish of shining, shimmering, grand-tasting good-for-you Jell-O! That ought to keep you happy." This is true; sugars' effects on neurotransmitters are pacifying. While these midcentury parents were wiser about protein, fats, organ meats, and fruits and vegetables (over grains), they were already making the mistake of using sugar to calm their babies and "make them happy."

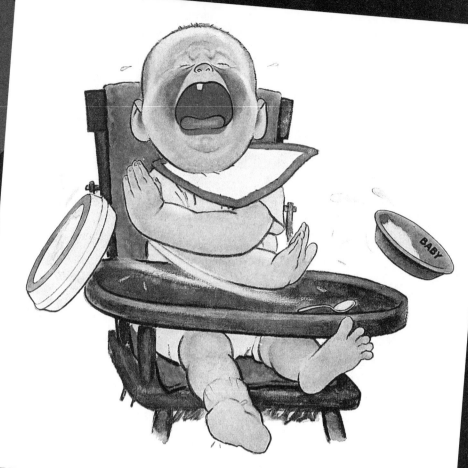

Now's the time for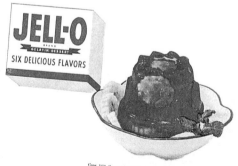

Hey, take it easy, Junior! Here comes a big dish of shining, shimmering, grand-tasting, good-for-you Jell-O! That ought to keep you happy! And Mommy, too, because Jell-O gelatin desserts are so easy to prepare.

JELL-O IS A REGISTERED TRADE-MARK OF GENERAL FOODS CORP

Copr. 1952, General Foods Corp.

Sugar Is Just One of the Sugars

"Table sugar" isn't the only sugar. You can also count the following obvious and hidden sweeteners as "sugars" to the body since they all detract from nutrients and disrupt normal functioning:

• Fruit juice concentrate/concentrated fruit juice
• Raw sugar, brown sugar
• Cane juice, cane sugar
• Agave nectar
• High fructose corn syrup, corn syrup, corn sugar
• Dextrose, ribose, sucrose
• Maltitol, sorbitol, mannitol
• Store-bought juice
• White flour products (organic or not: pasta, bread, bagels, pretzels, crackers, cookies, doughnuts, cake, pie, etc.)

Refined Flour Is Sugar. Starches, like white flour and white rice, break down into sugar during digestion. Thus, to consume white flour, you might as well have cotton candy as far as the body is concerned. Kathleen DesMaisons, Ph.D., author of *Little Sugar Addicts*, warns: "Sugar sensitive children can react to refined carbohydrates as if they were sugars." So when you think pretzels, sandwich bread, crackers, pancakes, and bagels are an okay, healthy, "low-fat" snack for your child, we beseech you to reconsider and recognize them as the "sweets" they are.

However, it is now known that fructose (previously thought of as a harmless "fruit sugar") also negatively affects insulin!

In addition to its effect on insulin, fructose damages the liver. The liver processes fructose in a way that's similar to how it processes alcohol; too much fructose results in fatty liver disease—a disorder commonly seen in alcoholics.

Alongside this rise in fructose (and overall sugar) consumption is a steep rise in heart disease, obesity, diabetes, cancer, and other 3Cs *in children*. With the known dietary dangers of glucose and a new, better understanding of how fructose harms health, it is logical that sugar plays a major role in chronic disease in both children and adults today. Dr. Lustig warns, "high-fructose corn syrup and sucrose are . . . *both poison in high doses*."

SUGAR HINDERS IMMUNITY

In addition to its druglike effects on mood and emotions, its disruption to the endocrine system, and its toxic effects on the liver, sugar is guilty of weakening the immune system. Studies show that the immune system's key white blood cells are *crippled* by sugar for 4 to 6 hours after sugar has been eaten. This means that if your child has just had some candy before a playdate and then is exposed to strep or a virus during it, she's much less able to defend herself. That is to say, she is more likely to get sick because she's consumed sugar. Further, sugar depletes B vitamins and other nutrients, which are critical to immune system functioning and protection against infection. Worse, sugar displaces more nutrient-dense foods in the diet, further reducing intake of nutrients that could protect her and strengthen her immunity.

SUGAR IS NOT NUTRIENT WORTHY

Russell L. Blaylock, M.D., neurosurgeon, author, excitotoxin expert, and nutrition researcher, states, "Sugar is the biggest enemy we face in the world of nutrition and health." Yet sugar is becoming an increasingly large part of our diet, although it offers no nutrition. The vitamins and minerals required to assimilate and digest it are absent, and so the body must donate from its stores of nutrients whenever sugar is eaten. Thus, sugar serves to deplete nutritional status and therefore diminishes health each time it is consumed.

Even in "moderation," sugar:
- Falsely stimulates appetite
- Causes inflammation
- Causes tooth decay
- Cripples your child's immune system for hours
- Disturbs calcium and magnesium metabolism
- Causes out-of-control behavior
- Elicits cravings for druglike effects—possibly laying the path for future alcohol and drug addiction
- Feeds yeast, disrupting healthy bacteria in the gut, causing the gut to be leaky
- Feeds cancer
- Creates critical mineral imbalances
- Depletes nutrients such as B vitamins, zinc, chromium, and magnesium
- Reduces the body's ability to detoxify
- Inhibits proper enzyme function
- Predisposes food allergies (particularly to foods eaten with it)
- Fattens the body and the blood
- Worsens heart health
- Causes emotional instability
- Disrupts hormones and neurotransmitters
- Disrupts the endocrine system, increasing the risk of diabetes and metabolic syndrome
- Hastens aging

One of sugar's worst offenses is robbing the body of nutrients, but that's not the *only* one. According to expert sugar researcher Nancy Appleton, Ph.D., author of the best-selling book *Lick the Sugar Habit*, it has nearly 150 ways of causing disease and dysfunction. Known as an antinutrient, sugar is best classified as a chemical, drug, or poison.

Sugar tears down each of the four pillars of Super Nutrition and must be seen as a serious threat to health: a digestive disrupter, a toxin, an immunity blocker, and a nutrient thief. *Every* bite of sugar brings with it serious health risks. Truly, sugar consumption should always be weighed against its risks.

Obesity and Diabetes

The CDC declares that childhood obesity has tripled in the last three decades, and that type 2 diabetes (formerly "adult-onset" diabetes) is a "sizable and growing problem among U.S. children."

Although both diabetes and obesity are associated with high sugar intake, common advice on how to combat diabetes and obesity has *not* been about lowering sugar, but rather on making diets lower and lower in *fat* and calories.

Despite this nearly universal low-fat focus, everyone is getting fatter. Even preschoolers: 15 percent are now overweight, double the number just twenty years ago. Kids today, though, are not "overnourished," nor do they have "too much nutrition"; rather, they are simply overstuffed with empty calories from too much white flour and sugar. *Since the advent of the low-fat diet and thousands of "low-fat" foods, we are fatter and more diabetic than ever—and so are our children.*

Food Abundance Doesn't Equal Nutrient Abundance!

Most people probably wouldn't consider U.S. children to be at similar risk for nutrient deficiencies as children in underdeveloped countries. Yet American children do have many common nutrient deficiencies that put their health at risk, despite many being overweight. When fed "empty" calories, the body is overfed but undernourished.

William Sears, M.D., in *The NDD™* (Nutrient Deficit Disorder) *Book*, warns that American children (regardless of their weight) are most commonly deficient in omega-3 fats, iron, zinc, magnesium, iodine, calcium, and vitamins B12, C, and E. Additionally, deficiencies in the fat-soluble vitamins D3 (upward of 80 percent), K2, and A are significant problems as well.

Lack of these nutrients leads to the following:
- Lowered immunity and susceptibility to pathogens
- Increased vulnerability to the impact of dietary and environmental toxins
- Increased activity of carcinogens, dietary opiates, and pathogenic flora

This increases risk for all 3C conditions.

Mother Nature doesn't ever provide calories without nutrients, but modern, man-made food is filled with such dietary abominations. *It is a new and bizarre phenomenon to be simultaneously overfed and undernourished.* Such calorie-rich, nutrient-poor diets are the crux of the 3C conditions.

The trends for increasing obesity and diabetes in children are going nowhere but up. Currently, it is estimated that over 30 percent of babies will develop diabetes and close to 50 percent will be overweight or obese. Cutting fat has obviously not been the solution. Experts, like Joseph Levy, M.D., professor of clinical pediatrics at Columbia University Medical Center in New York City, now clearly acknowledge *carbohydrates*—particularly refined flour and sugar—as being responsible for people being fat, countermanding the old dictates that fat was at fault. Dr. Levy states, "Many studies have confirmed that the liberal intake of carbohydrate is a major contributor to obesity."

When fat is removed to make "low-fat" or "fat-free" foods, the food doesn't taste good, so sugar and chemicals are added for flavor and preservation. No one tells you that sugar turns into body fat *easier* than dietary fat turns into body fat.

An Outdated Notion: All Calories Are *Not* Equal

We've all heard it: "A calorie is a calorie is a calorie." Weight loss is a simple formula, as if the body were just a machine: You must burn more calories than you take in. It doesn't really matter what food you eat—caloric intake and output determine weight. However, this is an old and oversimplified view of how food works in the body.

Food is far more than just calories. Elizabeth Lipski, Ph.D., C.C.N., clinical nutritionist and author of *Digestive Wellness for Children*, explains that "Food is *information* for our bodies and brains." Depending on the food, different neurotransmitters, hormones, and cellular messages are stimulated. The body "reads" food and does different things with it depending on what it is, how much energy and nutrients it provides, and what the current needs of the body happen to be. Foods that contain glucose and fructose, for example, send messages that trigger both fat storage and hunger more than other foods, says Robert Lustig, M.D., a pediatric neuroendocrinologist and professor.

Prevent Diabetes and Obesity with Super Nutrition

There's no way to sugarcoat it: Sugar makes people sick and fat, and sugar is far worse than fat when it comes to harming health. Here are some things you can do to protect your child against sugar's harmful effects.

Make sure gut flora is on track. Studies demonstrate that the kind of intestinal flora in the body can influence metabolism and appetite and therefore contribute to metabolic disorders like diabetes and obesity. Associate professor at Emory School of Medicine, Andrew Gerwitz, Ph.D., showed that simply transplanting the gut flora of obese mice into skinny mice made the skinny mice fat too. This means that what kind of gut flora you have impacts weight and even eating habits. Optimize your toddler's gut ecosystem by keeping sugar out of her diet because sugar feeds yeasts (which are fungi) and causes gut dysbiosis. Include lacto-fermented foods, fresh and cultured dairy, and probiotic supplements to help her intestinal health.

Exercise for endocrine stabilization, not calorie burning. Sunlight, fresh air, and exercise are all elements of a normal childhood. Get your child active and outdoors. Movement is important, but *not* for burning calories. Such activities are critical because they have a positive *hormonal* impact: they increase insulin sensitivity (the opposite of disease-related insulin resistance), and for that, they are protective against obesity and 3C conditions. Furthermore, physical movement and activity also naturally stimulate happiness neurotransmitters, making sugars less appealing.

Avoid the all-carbohydrate trap. Children's diets often tend to be all carbohydrate—grains and fruit, with some vegetables. Such carbohydrates tend to be fastest and most convenient, creating an "all-carb trap" for parents to fall into all too easily. Processed grains—chips, pretzels, bars, cereal—are especially easy to eat in isolation. It is important to ensure either animal protein or animal fats, or both, are part of every meal. Truly "balanced" meals are not based on grains; they are based on the presence of animal foods, with properly prepared carbohydrate foods and other whole foods as garnishes, digestive aids, and nutrient boosters.

Time to Stop Nursing or Bottle Feeding?

If you are still nursing at 12 months, we salute you (and hopefully your baby will thank you someday). Though it can be a rewarding experience for you and your baby, we know that breast-feeding can present evolving challenges such as teething (and biting!), countless distractions, and increasingly busy schedules. Further, social pressures are prevalent, and sadly many people feel it is excessive to nurse a baby beyond one year of age.

But what our modern society has forgotten is that your baby's sucking instinct goes beyond 12 months, lasting *at least* until she's 2½, as anthropological and infant-care research has shown. Both breast and bottle satisfy this suckling instinct. Completely weaning (or stopping nursing or the bottle altogether) leaves your baby without a way to satisfy this instinct. Furthermore, babies fully weaned from mom's milk get sick more often since they're no longer receiving the living immune-boosting factors that come with it.

Continuing to nurse beyond one year provides benefits to both mom and baby:

▸ Immune support—shortening the duration and lessening the frequency and severity of illness
▸ Perfect nutrition for your baby
▸ Fewer orthodontic problems
▸ Allergy prevention
▸ Continued bond and comforting mechanism
▸ An ability to provide hydration and nutrition during illness
▸ Earlier reading in boys and fewer speech problems
▸ A natural way to space pregnancies
▸ Calorie burning for mom
▸ Calming and loving hormones for mom and baby, resulting in reduced stress and anxiety for both
▸ Reduced breast cancer and rheumatoid arthritis risk for mom—the longer you nurse, the better the protection

So our advice on weaning is not to, just yet. When it is time to wean (which you'll realize as your child is less interested in nursing and as feedings are gradually skipped or missed), there are ways to best protect and ensure your baby's health during and after the transition to end nursing.

Because your baby's gut flora changes as she weans, it is of utmost importance to continue providing good probiotics to your baby during this time. Sources of probiotics include lacto-fermented foods and raw and cultured dairy. If you are not providing such foods, then giving a daily probiotic supplement is helpful (typically a small dose once or twice a day is adequate, according to the directions on the bottle). Additionally, once nursing has stopped, there are benefits to having a stored supply of breast milk in your freezer, especially for times when your child gets sick and is in need of an immune boost. Stored milk is also helpful for softening the impact of the cow's milk on the gut since you can intersperse your milk with the newly introduced cow's milk. Furthermore, whey can be made from pumped milk (see Mommy Whey, page 64) and stored for 2 to 3 months. This whey can then be used for lacto-fermenting foods for your baby, enabling her to continue to benefit from your milk both from its nutrients and from lacto-fermentation.

To ease the transition on your child, one gentle weaning method is to avoid offering the breast or bottle, but not to refuse when your child asks. Slowly begin to delay or distract your child when she indicates she wants to nurse or have a bottle, which will gradually lead to skipped feedings. Over 3 to 4 weeks, your milk supply will begin to diminish. According to William Sears, M.D., removing a feeding every 3 to 7 days is about as fast as is wise to wean—much faster, and you increase your chance of developing mastitis.

Protect Your Child with Natural Nourishment

The typical diet for a 12- to 18-month-old baby often includes pasteurized cheese cubes, sugared cereals, juice boxes, pasteurized milk, sweetened flavored yogurt, crackers, cookies, pasta, microwavable toddler meals, teething biscuits or puffs, and "fruit" snacks.

Low in fat and high in sugar, such typical toddler foods supply chemicals, antinutrients, allergens, and toxins, but what they do not supply is sufficient nutrition. There is a better diet for your 12- to 18-month-old. It includes natural fat, "wise" carbs, even smarter sweets, and appropriate "big-kid" beverages.

USE FAT FOR FUEL

Fat is the best basis of energy for children. Benefits of a fat-based diet include the following:

▸ Stimulating leptin, sending "I'm-full" messages and reducing overeating
▸ Ensuring fat-soluble antioxidants, vitamins, and mineral activators will be absorbed
▸ Having antimicrobial, antiviral, and immune-supportive factors
▸ Keeping blood sugar balanced
▸ Helping intestinal function and slowing down digestion so more nutrients can be absorbed
▸ Providing nutrition for your toddler's growing, developing brain
▸ Promoting healthy skin and cells
▸ Making foods delicious!

Let your child enjoy butter on veggies and grains, whole milk, full-fat yogurt, red meat, and dark-meat poultry with the skin. When the diet is purely traditional foods, fat need not be feared but appreciated for its nutritional value and health benefits.

BE WISE WITHIN THE WORLD OF CARBOHYDRATES

As your baby's carbohydrate world widens with the introduction of greens, nuts, and more raw veggies, we have some cautions. We recommend *most* carbohydrate foods be veggies and greens, with fewer coming from starchy veggies and nuts and even fewer from seeds, tubers, and tropical fruits. Fewer still should come from grains and legumes, with fewest from whole-foods sweeteners. Within these categories of plant foods, be varied. Of the 50,000 edible plant foods on the planet, only fifteen crops provide 90 percent of the world's food, and just three make up *60 percent* of the caloric intake of the world: rice, corn, and wheat. But Nature provides many more options than the rice cakes, corn chips, and wheat-based crackers, cookies, and bars in the grocery store's center aisles.

A BETTER WAY TO SOOTHE THE SWEET-TOOTH MONSTER

Here are tips on avoiding refined sugars in your child's diet and how to incorporate naturally sweet *whole foods* that are less deleterious to nutritional status than processed, refined sugars.

Don't introduce refined sugars. Without the experience of the druglike taste and psychotropic effects of refined sugars, children will adore Nature's sweeteners and will never feel deprived or wanting. For the first several years, you are in control of your child's diet, and there is no need to have refined sugar. Further, Dr. Lipski points out that children's "digestive systems cannot handle . . . sugars other than lactose until the age of three."

Use whole-foods sweeteners. Sweets that come from Nature in whole form will not only be pleasing to the palate, but they will actually provide nutrients as well. Often natural sweeteners contain nutrients that help glucose tolerance and sugar metabolism, such as chromium, magnesium, and B vitamins. Natural sweeteners include grade B maple syrup, whole plant stevia, and raw honey, as well as those listed on page 182.

Use even the natural sweets sparingly. Be discerning when you decide what calls for an out-of-the-ordinary sweet treat, offering whole fruit on a daily basis for meeting the "sweet" needs of the taste buds. Reserve any concentrated sweets (even from whole foods) for special occasions.

Consume with controllers. Fats and protein reduce the impact of skyrocketing blood sugar and insulin that result when sweets are eaten untempered. Keeping blood sugar steady is ideal for overall health, metabolic stability, and emotional, behavioral consistency. Providing plenty of fat and protein, along with carbs that naturally contain fiber, helps to temper the sugar spike. And omega-3 fats in cod liver oil and fats from grass-fed animal foods (like butter) are good examples of fats that help to improve insulin sensitivity.

Don't promote self-medicating with sugars. We agree with Dr. William Sears, author of more than forty books on child care, who advises: "I've seen so many parents comfort a crying child by saying, 'Here, have a drink of your soda' or 'Have a bite of your cookie' to make him feel better. . . . [which] gives children a terrible message about eating food for emotional rather than nutritional reasons. When your children feel sad, give them a hug and a smile. It's better for them!" We urge you not to build the association with food, particularly sugary foods, as solace or reward.

NATURAL AND NUTRITIOUS BIG-KID BEVERAGES

"Typical" dietary changes at age one include switching your baby from formula to pasteurized cow's milk and often mark the end of nursing or bottle feeding, too.

But cow's milk isn't all it's campaigned to be. As we described in chapter 1, pasteurized milk is highly processed and is a source of allergens, toxins, denatured proteins, less-absorbable calcium and minerals, and reduced vitamins. Far from a natural nourishing food, it can cause intestinal bleeding and is linked to autoimmune disease development.

Say "no" to bean, grain, seed, and nut "milks." For those with an allergy or intolerance to processed cow's milk, new alternative "milks" are available. However, soy, rice, hemp, and almond milk are poor substitutes for human milk or homemade formula based on their low nutrient value, low fat content, synthetic nutrients, degree of processing, and the various sweeteners and additives that increase palatability and texture. Even coconut milk, though great for recipes, isn't sufficient as a replacement for mom's milk after complete weaning.

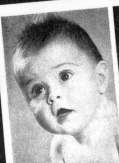
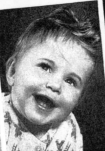
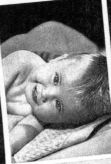
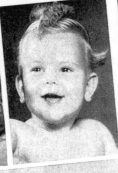

Rx For Happy Feeding in Listless Weather:

SERVE YOUR BABY THESE MAIN-DISH FOODS

—combinations of all the meat, all the vegetables Baby needs

In hot weather, Baby's appetite may lag. How important, then, for the foods he does eat to be extra-nourishing. Campbell's Baby Soups are just that. They offer the latest advance in baby feeding . . . meat and vegetables *in combination*.

Baby needs meat. These main-dish foods give him meat. He needs vegetables and cereal. He gets them here. All the meat . . . all the vegetables a growing, happy baby requires. And how convenient! Baby's main dish from just one glass jar!

Four different meats that doctors recommend . . . beef, chicken, liver, lamb . . . are combined with tender vegetables and cereal. Then there's an all-vegetable soup of eight vegetables and oatmeal. All five of firm, strained-food consistency.

Serve these five, in turn, as Baby's substantial main dish. Here's a sound, well-rounded feeding plan for Baby . . . and less work for you.

Hints on Summer Feeding

● Small baby, big thirst . . . so offer water freely between meals.

● Babies take to these main-dish foods. They taste better, mothers say.

● Can be fed as early as any strained foods. Ask your doctor "when?" and "how much?"

● Every grocer who sells Campbell's Soups can supply Campbell's Baby Soups.

Campbell's STRAINED **BABY SOUPS**
Main-dish foods for Baby

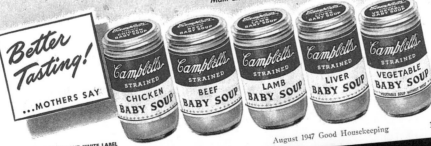

Better Tasting! . . . MOTHERS SAY

LOOK FOR THE RED-AND-WHITE LABEL

August 1947 Good Housekeeping

115

Instead of processed drinks, choose a beverage with "benefits" (those that follow). Of course, if you're still nursing, your milk is the *best* beverage for your baby—preferably from the breast, but even expressed in a cup at this age is preferred over any other beverage.

Lacto-fermented beverages and other healthful drinks. Lacto-fermented beverages include Pretty Pink Drink (beet kvass, page 114), coconut kefir (from coconut water or coconut milk, page 112) and homemade recipes for ginger ale, apple cider, and homemade orangina (see recipes in this chapter). Souper Stock can always be used as a nutritious beverage, as can coconut water; and for additional, occasional beverages, we recommend the excellent book *Nourishing Traditions* by Sally Fallon for more recipes—including homemade rice milk and almond drink.

Real milk. Far better than factory-farmed, processed, pasteurized, homogenized milk is *real milk*. Real, unpasteurized, raw milk from cows or goats eating grass out on pasture is the ideal weaning beverage for your child. This milk is also designed to optimally nourish babies and is surprisingly similar to human milk (see table), as it is a living food with ideal immune constituents, vitamins, minerals, probiotics, and enzymes.

Recipes That Say Sayonara to Sugar

Your baby's carbohydrate-digestion capabilities are improving. Thus, she can now handle some raw veggies and uncooked nontropical fruits, as well as a few starches. Enzymes from mom's milk or homemade formula; raw and cultured dairy; lacto-fermented fruits, veggies, and beverages; and Souper Stock all aid digestion, so don't stop feeding these to her.

FEEDING AT 12 TO 15 MONTHS

Between 12 and 15 months, you can introduce whole eggs, honey, tomato, citrus fruits, some very limited natural sweeteners, cooked leafy greens, and liverwurst. For a more complete list of acceptable foods at this age, see the Food Introduction Timeline on page 222.

Pattern	12 to 18 months
Early AM	Early morning nursing and breakfast
Mid-Morning	Snack and possibly nursing
Mid-Day	Meal
Afternoon	Nursing or bottle (before nap)
Evening	Meal
Nighttime	Nursing or bottle (before bed)

Comparing the Many Forms of Milk from Fresh to Highly Processed

Note that commercial infant formula, made from pasteurized and highly processed cow's milk,
is also lacking in the living factors so plentiful and nourishing in raw milk from humans and cows.

Nutrients & Immune Factors	Raw Mom's Milk	Raw Cow's Milk	Pasteurized Cow's Milk	Commercial Infant Formula
Anti-microbial enzymes	Active	Active	Inhabited	Unavailable
Biodiverse probiotics	Active	Active	Destroyed	Added
Essential fatty acids	Active	Active	Damaged	Added
Lactase-producing bacteria	Active	Active	Destroyed	Unavailable
Delicate proteins	Active	Active	Destroyed	Altered
B-12 biding proteins	Active	Active	Inactive	Inactive
Bioavailable vitamins	Active	Active	Inhabited	Inhibited
Bioavailable calcium	Active	Active	Inhabited	Inhibited
Bioavailable phosphorus	Active	Active	Inhabited	Inhibited
Phosphatase enzyme	Active	Active	Destroyed	Inhibited
Oligosaccharides	Active	Active	Diminished	Unavailable
Lymphocytes	Active	Active	Inactive	Unavailable
B-lymphocytes	Active	Active	Inactive	Inactive
Macrophages	Active	Active	Inactive	Inactive
Neutrophils	Active	Active	Inactive	Inactive
IgA/IgG Antibodies	Active	Active	Inactive	Inactive
Gamma-interferon	Active	Active	Inactive	Inactive
Fibronectin	Active	Active	Inactive	Inactive

Courtesy of The Weston A. Price Foundation. Reprinted with permission.

Super Nutrition Food Categorizations for 12 to 18 Months

Super POWER	PURE
Anchovies, sardines	Organic fruits and veggies
Lacto-fermented beverages and sides	Organic, free-range eggs
Liverwurst	Organic, pastured meats
Raw dairy	

OKAY	CRAP
Fruits/veggies, washed nonorganic	Rice cakes
Nonorganic trim meats	Fishie crackers, teddy cookies, cereal, candy
Nonorganic eggs	Juice (even 100 percent organic)
Nonorganic butter	

Creamed Spinach

Uncooked spinach is inappropriate for a baby this age (as are other raw leafy greens), as it contains oxalic acid (oxalates) that blocks calcium and iron absorption and irritates the mouth and intestinal tract. Cooking helps to neutralize much of the oxalic acid, so any spinach served to your baby must be well cooked.

1 bag chopped spinach

2 tablespoons (28 g) butter

1 clove minced garlic

¼ small onion, finely chopped

⅓ cup (80 ml) heavy cream (preferably farm fresh, but not ultrapasteurized)

⅓ cup (33 g) freshly grated (preferably raw) Parmesan cheese

In a skillet, heat the spinach on medium-low, stirring constantly until wilted. Remove the spinach from the skillet, drain, and squeeze out any water.

Add the butter to the warm skillet. When it is melted, add the garlic and onion. Sauté and stir for 3 to 5 minutes.

Reintroduce the spinach to the skillet and slowly mix in the cream.

Slowly sprinkle the Parmesan over the top. Continue to stir until the cheese is melted.

Yield: 1 to 2 baby and 1 to 2 adult servings

Liverwurst

Liverwurst is a most nutritious convenience food. Because unhealthy liver can contain toxins, it is of paramount importance to get clean liver. We've found the very best quality and taste comes from www.uswellnessmeats.com, from which liverwurst comes frozen. Place it in the refrigerator for 24 hours to thaw. (Eat within 1 week of defrosting.) Slice and serve! It tastes great with sliced avocado and perhaps even some mustard. Liverwurst is a great on-the-go snack with a small cooler pack.

Mom to Mom / Offer no grains until at least 1 year of age, ideally 18 months. When you include grains, they should be whole (not refined, bleached, or enriched) and should ideally be gluten-free (not wheat, rye, or barley just yet). Grains should also always be sprouted or soaked. Limit crackers, cereal, teething biscuits, bagels, or toast.

Berries Parfait with Cinnamon Sprinkle

Your baby can now eat uncooked berries. To create a parfait, combine ½ cup (115 g) yogurt (preferably raw, plain, whole, grass-fed, organic) with cinnamon (which is known to improve glucose tolerance). Then alternately layer with blueberries, raspberries, and finely chopped strawberries. Top this lovely parfait with farm-fresh cream, if desired.

Citrus Fruit Splash Salad

For a tart treat you can feed your tiny toddler for dessert, combine chopped grapefruit, orange, and strawberries. Add a squeeze of lemon or lime juice and a splash of kombucha (see page 185).

Quiche

Quiche is an excellent food for breakfast, lunch, or dinner. Traditionally it uses a white flour crust, but in this variation, we use coconut flour and arrowroot starch, which is naturally white, not refined. It has been found to be very digestible, even by babies.

½ cup (64 g) arrowroot starch

½ cup (56 g) coconut flour

2 tablespoons (30 g) plain yogurt

½ cup (120 ml) water

Stir all ingredients together in a covered glass bowl and leave on the counter to soak overnight.

For Crust:

¼ cup (52 g) room-temperature lard

¼ cup (55 g) room-temperature butter

½ cup (43 g) coconut, shredded, unsweetened, unsulfured

¼ teaspoons Celtic sea salt

In a large bowl, mix together the flour, salt, and the fats. Spread evenly in 2 pie plates to make thin-bottom crusts. Bake at 350°F (180°C, gas mark 4) for 10 to 15 minutes.

For Filling:

6 eggs

1 cup (235 ml) milk

¼ cup (60 ml) fresh cream

½ to ¾ cup (58 to 86 g) shredded cheese

½ cup (about 70 g) precooked meat (bacon, leftover chicken, or chopped organic ham lunch meat)

1 cup (71 g) broccoli florets

Mix all ingredients together. Pour half of the mixed filling into each crust. Bake for 45 to 55 minutes at 350°F (180°C, gas mark 4) or until a knife inserted into the center of each quiche comes out clean.

Yield: 2 quiches

Notes

• Read more about soaking ingredients in chapter 6.
• *Soufflé variation:* Skip crust and separate the egg whites, whipping them into stiff peaks and adding them last, just before baking.
• *Muffin variation:* Skip the crust and pour the egg filling mixture into 24 muffin tins lined with cupcake liners.

The Real Deal Fishie Snacks

These small sea treasures are rich in omega-3 oils and low in toxins since they are low on the food chain. Often, the whole anchovy is eaten—bones, organs, and all—creating one of the best "whole foods" available. Puree the whole fish (along with olive oil they are packed in) with a blender or food processor, ensuring all bones are fully ground before spoon feeding to your baby. You can find dehydrated anchovies at www.radiantlifecatalog.com; these are quick, easy, on-the-go treats that your baby will enjoy alone or mixed into other foods. They are extremely nutritious because they are well preserved through the process of drying. Crumble the dried fish into other meals to give a Super POWER nutrition boost.

Beets and Peaches Salad

This recipe is adapted from From Asparagus to Zucchini, *published by the Madison Area Community Supported Agriculture Coalition.*

½ pound (225 g) finely diced, washed beets

1 peach

For Vinaigrette:

1 clove minced garlic

Celtic sea salt (¼ teaspoon or to taste)

1 tablespoon (15 ml) olive oil

1 tablespoon (15 ml) raw apple cider vinegar

½ teaspoon grated gingerroot, optional

⅓ cup (42 g) raspberries, optional

Juice of half an orange, freshly squeezed, optional

Roast the beets on a cookie sheet or in a roasting pan for 45 minutes at 350°F (180°C, gas mark 4). Allow to cool. Peel and dice the peach and add it to the beets.

To make the vinaigrette, mix the garlic, salt, olive oil, vinegar, and ginger in a small bowl. Pour over the beets and peaches.

Optional: Add raspberries, ginger, and orange juice.

Note

- The recipe works best if allowed to marinate, but it can also be served immediately.

Yield: 4 servings for baby

Cod Liver Oil

Cod liver oil was discussed in chapter 4. Now that your baby is one year old, you can increase the dosage to 1 teaspoon of high quality or ½ teaspoon fermented. See Resources, page 218, for preferred brands.

Marinade for Aging Beef

Aged beef, as you find it at www.uswellnessmeats.com, is "predigested." It is easier on your baby's digestive system, more tender, and more flavorful. If aged meat is not available, instead marinate your meat to tenderize and thus make it more digestible. Marinating is also protective against carcinogens when barbecuing meat. Mix high-quality, cold-pressed olive oil and fresh herbs and spices with some raw apple cider vinegar. Cover meat with marinade and let soak for 12 hours in the refrigerator. One hour before cooking, take the meat out of the refrigerator and allow it to warm to room temperature. Cook as desired.

Gingerbread Man Milkshake

This is a great "dessert" for a special occasion or holiday. The benefit of raw or rare animal foods is their unadulterated state of nutrition (undamaged vitamins and minerals), but they're most beneficial due to their enzyme content (enzymes are destroyed by cooking). Experts in traditional-foods nutrition and the health benefits that can be expected highlight that such a diet must always contain some raw animal foods (such as raw milk or raw eggs in just such a recipe as this).

½ cup (115 g) yogurt

¼ cup (60 ml) fresh, raw milk

1 teaspoon blackstrap molasses

½ teaspoon freshly grated ginger (or ¼ teaspoon powdered)

½ teaspoon ground cinnamon

½ small brown spotted banana

Egg yolk, optional

In a blender, combine the yogurt, milk, molasses, ginger, cinnamon, and banana. Add the egg yolk, if using.

Yield: ¾ cup (175 ml) (closer to 1 cup or 235 ml with banana)

Notes

- If you use a raw egg yolk, choose a farm-fresh, pastured egg (if you'd rather, or have store-bought lower-quality eggs, boil the egg for 3.5 minutes and use this yolk). The yolk adds important amino acids and protein, making this smoothie a complete meal, as well as omega-3 fats and various other vitamins and minerals. Most of all, a raw or rare yolk adds a very significant amount of enzymes to the meal.
- Coconut milk or kefir can replace the dairy milk.
- Milkshake ingredients can also include coconut flour, freshly ground flaxseed, raw honey, or dates.
- Ginger can be "spicy"—start with less and add more as your baby gets used to it.

Apple-Pear Compote

This is a great fall treat after a cool afternoon outside gathering leaves.

3 tablespoons (42 g) butter, ghee, or coconut oil

2 apples chopped into bite sizes for your baby

2 pears chopped into bite sizes for your baby

½ teaspoon ground cinnamon

½ teaspoon ground nutmeg

½ teaspoon ground allspice

1 teaspoon vanilla extract

2 tablespoons (18 g) organic raisins or finely chopped dried dates or figs, optional

In a skillet, warm the fat on medium-low. Add the apples and pears to the skillet. Sprinkle in all the spices. Pour in the vanilla. Add the optional dried fruit and stir until the fruit softens. This recipe is best served warm.

Yield: About 1 quart (950 ml)

Sausage Cheeseballs and Savory Sauce

These are kid-tested favorites.

½ pound (225 g) ground sausage (or plain ground pork, then add seasonings and sea salt)

½ pound (225 g) ground beef (with heart, if available)

1 egg

¼ cup (28 g) coconut flour or arrowroot starch

Sprinkle of cayenne or red pepper

1 teaspoon Celtic sea salt (more if using bulk pork instead of sausage)

½ cup (60 g) grated cheese (any kind, preferably raw)

For Sauce:

2 tablespoons (28 g) butter, ghee, coconut oil, or (26 g) lard

1 clove minced garlic

¼ small onion, finely chopped

1 large tomato, sliced or chopped

½ teaspoon oregano

½ teaspoon basil

1 teaspoon Celtic sea salt

½ cup (120 ml) previously made Souper Stock

In a large bowl, mix together the sausage and ground beef. Add the egg, arrowroot starch, cayenne, salt, and cheese. Knead all ingredients together and form into 1-inch (2.5 cm) balls. In a large skillet, sauté in warmed lard or coconut oil, turning frequently on all sides on medium.

To make the sauce, in a separate saucepan, warm the fat over medium heat and add the garlic and onion. Sauté for

3 to 5 minutes. Add the chopped tomato, oregano, basil, and salt. Add the Souper Stock and stir occasionally for 10 to 15 minutes.

Let the sausage balls cool. Cut them into bite-size chunks and drizzle them with the tomato sauce.

Yield: 2 adult servings and 1 for baby

Note

• Meatloaf Muffins (variation): Use 1 pound (455 g) ground beef (with heart, if available). Add a mixed seasoning with oregano and add basil to taste. Include 1 clove minced garlic and 1 small diced tomato. Place the mixture in lined muffin tins. Bake at 325°F (170°C, gas mark 3) for 15 to 20 minutes.

FEEDING AT 15 TO 18 MONTHS

Between 15 and 18 months, you can introduce soaked and sprouted nuts and seeds, lacto-fermented beverages, a few more raw veggies, and limited carob. For a more complete list of acceptable foods at this age, see the Food Introduction Timeline on page 222.

Soaked and Sprouted Nuts and Seeds

Sprouting nuts and seeds makes them much more digestible and nutritious. After nuts and seeds are sprouted and dried, they can be ground into flour for recipes. For nuts, try pecans, almonds, or walnuts (these are different from peanuts, which are not actually nuts, but legumes). For seeds, try pumpkin, squash, sunflower, and

sesame. New research suggests that delaying introduction of nuts increases the risk of nut allergies. To actually reduce the likelihood that your baby develops allergies, soaking or sprouting nuts and seeds is strongly suggested. (See "Create Carb Safety," page 146.)

Soaked Nuts

Nuts (pecans, almonds, walnuts, or others)
Water (twice as much as quantity of nuts)
1 to 2 tablespoons (15 to 30 g) Celtic sea salt

Soak the nuts in water with salt for 12 to 24 hours, covered. Rinse well. Dry the nuts on cookie sheets lined with paper towels, switching the paper towels throughout the day; alternatively dry in a warm oven (150°F [66°C] or the lowest setting on your oven) or use a dehydrator (the best and easiest option).

Notes

• This same process can be applied to seeds.

Sprouted Nuts and Seeds

Soak nuts or seeds in twice as much water as nuts and 1 to 2 tablespoons (15 to 30 g) sea salt. Cover for 12 hours. Rinse and drain every 3 to 4 hours or just leave the mixture overnight. Rinse very well.

Place the seeds or nuts in a jar (find a sprouting jar at your health food store or online).

If you do not have a sprouting jar, secure cheesecloth over the top of a Mason jar with a rubber band. Angle the jar, top down, in a dish-draining rack. Every 6 to 8 hours rinse 2 or 3 times by filling the jar with water and shaking, then draining.

When you notice sprouts (more obvious with seeds), move the jar into a well-lit area (but not direct sunlight) and continue to rinse well every 6 to 8 hours. Let sprouts grow for 3 to 5 days until you actually see a small sprout appear (be cautious during rinsing not to break it off, as this will cause spoiling during the sprouting process).

When complete, rinse very well. Dry on cookie sheets lined with paper towels, switching the paper towel throughout the day; alternatively dry in a warm oven (150°F [66°C] or the lowest setting on your oven) or use a dehydrator (the best option).

Yield: Will be equal to the amount of nuts or seeds used; typically 2 to 3 cups (about 200 to 300 g)

Notes

- Well-dried sprouts and nuts and seeds can be stored in the refrigerator or cool pantry for 4 to 8 weeks.
- Sprouted nuts and seeds can be ground up and used as flour in many recipes or processed with additional oil into homemade nut or seed butters or spreads. The significance of sprouting is that the nutritional value has been increased, the digestibility improved, and the antinutrients minimized; the actual sprout itself isn't important.
- Brazil nuts, chestnuts, hazelnuts, pistachios, macadamia nuts, and pine nuts can also be used. Delay introducing peanuts until all other nuts have been introduced.
- Peanuts and cashews are actually legumes and shouldn't be soaked longer than 6 hours.

Apples and Nut Butter

Apples and pears have been cooked till now but can be consumed raw in small bites at this stage. Served with specially prepared nut butters, they make a nutritious and delicious snack.

Nut butters like almond, sunflower seed, and cashew can be purchased, but since those were not previously soaked, homemade is better. (Soaking is far easier and less time intensive than sprouting.)

Nut Flour or Seed Flour

Grind presoaked, dried nuts or seeds in a food processor or a coffee grinder.

Nut Butter

2 cups (about 200 g) soaked and dried nuts

¼ teaspoon Celtic sea salt, or more to taste

2 tablespoons (28 ml or 28 g) oil (almond, coconut, or other)

½ teaspoon almond extract, optional

In a food processor or Vitamix, mix together the nuts, salt, optional almond extract, and oil. Grind well. Store in the refrigerator in a mason jar. Serve rolled into balls.

Yield: 1¼ cups (about 325 g) nut butter

Zucchini Banana Bread

What a delicious bread this is for a healthy snack, well-buttered. Can also be dipped in beaten egg mixed with raw milk and cinnamon to make "French toast."

½ cup (64 g) arrowroot starch

½ cup (56 g) coconut flour

¾ cup (175 ml) water

1 tablespoon (15 g) yogurt

¾ cup (90 g) grated zucchini

1 tablespoon (14 g) butter

3 brown-spotted bananas

5 eggs

½ cup (115 g) yogurt

1 tablespoon (7 g) Bernard Jensen's gelatin, optional (www.radiantlifecatalog.com)

In a medium-size bowl, mix together the arrowroot starch, coconut flour, water, and yogurt. Soak overnight.

The next day, in a skillet, sauté the zucchini in butter. Purée the bananas with the eggs and stir in the yogurt. In a large bowl, mix with the presoaked flour mixture and the zucchini. Add the gelatin, if using.

Bake the mixture in a glazed ceramic loaf pan at 325°F (170°C, gas mark 6) for 25 to 35 minutes or until knife comes out clean from center.

Yield: 1 loaf

Variations

- Instead of zucchini and banana, use 1½ cups (368 g) baked sweet potato or baked pumpkin; add 2 teaspoons of pumpkin pie spice and ½ teaspoon vanilla.
- To bake pumpkin, slice it in half, scoop out the seeds, and place the halves face down in a pan filled with 1 inch (2.5 cm) of water for 45 minutes at 325°F (170°C, gas mark 3).
- This can optionally be made into muffins.

Doughnut Crepes

These crepes are a sweet treat, reminiscent of doughnuts in taste, though not in shape. They are particularly tasty when served topped with Apple or Pear Spread (page 161).

½ cup (64 g) arrowroot starch

2 eggs

2 egg whites

¼ teaspoon green powder stevia

Pinch Celtic sea salt

1 mashed, brown-spotted banana

2 tablespoons (30 g) yogurt

3 to 4 tablespoons (39 to 52 g) lard, (42 to 55 g) bacon grease, butter, or ghee

In a large bowl, combine the arrowroot starch, eggs, egg white, stevia, salt, banana, and yogurt.

Heat the fat over medium heat—¼ inch (0.5 cm) at least deep in hot pan.

Pour the batter into the pan and tip to spread the batter thinly over the bottom surface. When tiny bubbles appear or an edge lifts, flip crepe and cook on the other side for about 2 minutes.

Optional: For a very special treat—drizzle with maple syrup, raw honey, or sprinkle with Rapadura.

Yield: 6 to 8 crepes

Fish "Sticks" and Tartar Sauce

Free of preservatives, white flour, and flavor enhancers, homemade fish sticks are marvelous.

For Fish Sticks:

1 pound (455 g) cod or other deep-water fish, cut into strips or chunks

1 beaten egg

½ cup (about 50 g) grated cheese like parmesan, romano, or asiago (preferably raw)

(continued)

Choose Seafood Wisely

As our waters have become increasingly polluted, it is important to choose fish carefully. Monterey Bay Aquarium (www.montereybayaquarium.org, search "seafood watch") maintains a list of which seafood to buy or avoid, and the Environmental Defense Fund (www.edf.org, search for "seafood health alerts") suggests number of times certain fish can be eaten per month. Here are some general guidelines.

- The smaller the fish, the less toxic (sardines, anchovies, and fish roe are best) and can be eaten up to three times per week.

- The FDA warns pregnant and nursing moms to avoid shark, swordfish, king mackerel, and tilefish; we also suggest avoiding marlin, orange roughy, and big-eye or Ahi tuna.
- Lower-mercury seafood (salmon, shrimp, canned light tuna, pollock) can be consumed once per week, along with with clam, crab, flounder, herring, haddock, oysters, scallops, sole, and whitefish.
- Albacore tuna has significantly more mercury than "light" tuna, so should be avoided, as should Chilean sea bass, bluefish, and grouper.

¾ cup (96 g) arrowroot starch

1 teaspoon Celtic sea salt

1 teaspoon dill

3 to 4 tablespoons (42 to 55 g) butter or (39 to 52 g) lard

Dip the fish into the egg so it is coated on all sides. Place the other ingredients into a mason jar or large zip-top plastic bag. Add the fish to the jar or bag and shake to coat the fish. In a large skillet, sauté the coated fish in fat over medium heat, allowing each side to brown to golden for 3 to 5 minutes. Flip a few times during the cooking process.

For Tartar Sauce:

1 tablespoon (15 ml) unpasteurized pickle juice

½ cup (115 g) yogurt

1 tablespoon (15 ml) farm-fresh cream or whipping cream (not ultrapasteurized)

½ teaspoon dill

½ teaspoon Celtic sea salt

½ teaspoon mixed seasoning

Pinch of whole-plant ground stevia, optional

Mix all ingredients together in a medium-size bowl. Use to top warm fish.

Yield: 4 to 6 servings for baby

Birthday Bash without the Sugar Crash

Try this decadent carob brownie, served as cake, with optional banana cream cheese frosting. The brownie recipe is from Wholesome Home Cooking: Preparing Nutrient-Dense Foods.

1 cup (160 g) carob powder

1 cup (225 g) butter

¾ cup (255 g) honey, raw, unfiltered

4 eggs

1¼ cups (144 g) almond flour (see recipe for nut flour, page 137)

1 cup (80 g) walnuts, finely ground

2 teaspoons vanilla extract

In a large bowl, mix all ingredients together until lumps are no longer present. Bake for 30 minutes at 325°F (170°C, gas mark 3) in a 9 × 13 × 2-inch (23 × 33 × 5 cm) pan. Do not overbake.

Frosting

1 (8 oz. 225 g) package organic (preferably cultured) cream cheese or yogurt cheese (see recipe, page 92)

1 stick organic butter, softened

1 medium, brown spotted banana

Blend well with hand blender, Vitamix, or standing mixer. Spread over cooled brownie "cake."

BEVERAGES

The foremost authority on traditional-foods cuisine and health benefits is *Nourishing Traditions*, by Sally Fallon. From this excellent resource and "kitchen bible," we have provided you with several beverage options below, with permission.

Homemade Orangina

This is a favorite beverage for children in France, though the commercial form has excessive sugar. Making your own at home makes juice nutritious.

Juice of 12 oranges

2 teaspoons Celtic sea salt

¼ cup (60 ml) whey (see Homemade Whey, page 64)

½ teaspoon orange extract

1 ¼ quarts (1.2 L) filtered water

Place all ingredients in a 2-quart (1.9 L) jar. Stir well and cover tightly. Leave at room temperature for 48 hours and then move to the refrigerator. Stir before serving.

Yield: 2 quarts (1.9 L)

Mom to Mom / Though she can't speak well yet, your baby is intently listening. Repeatedly tell her what foods and beverages you are feeding her at each meal and snack. Eventually she'll have names for the foods she likes so that she can ask for them. Tell her about the food you are feeding her; she can understand far more than she can say.

Homemade Apple Cider

This takes many apples but is such a wonderful treat, especially in the autumn, it is well worth it!

24 organic apples

½ tablespoon (8 g) Celtic sea salt

¼ cup (60 ml) whey (see Homemade Whey, page 64)

Wash, peel, core, and quarter the apples. Process through a juicer. Remove foam. Strain the juice and stir in the sea salt and whey. Cover with cheesecloth and leave at room temperature for 72 hours. Skim off any foam and then place in Mason jars (two 2-quart [1.9 L] size).

It is ready to drink right away, but store it for a few weeks in the refrigerator as flavor develops.

Yield: ½ gallon (1.9 L)

Note

• This recipe requires a juicer or Vitamix.

> **Mom to Mom /** For those who are on a very tight budget, eggs are an excellent and affordable source of protein. Also, making Souper Stocks and soups is economical, since bones or chicken backs and fee are inexpensive. Organ meats and fattier muscle meats are often less expensive. Fats like lard are very inexpensive, and leftover bacon grease, schmaltz, or beef fat can be reused for other cooking that day or the next. Certainly, avoiding restaurant meals and sugary snack foods and drinks like juice and soda pop are budget savers as well.

Homemade Ginger Ale

Ginger is an excellent digestive aid that works great for nausea during pregnancy. This drink is the inspiration for the modern-day high fructose corn syrup–infused version.

¾ cup (96 g) fresh ginger, peeled and grated or chopped

½ cup (120 ml) fresh lime juice

¼ cup (48 g) Rapunzel brand Rapadura or other whole-foods sweetener

2 teaspoons Celtic sea salt

¼ cup (60 ml) whey (see Homemade Whey, page 64)

2 quarts (1.9 L) filtered water

Mix together all ingredients in a 2-quart (1.9 L) jug. Leave at room temperature for 48 to 72 hours and then move to the refrigerator. Strain into the glass when serving.

Yield: 2 quarts (1.9 L)

Notes

- This will keep for several months in the refrigerator.
- *Optional*: Mix with carbonated water.

Coconut Lime "Spritzer"

Juice of one lime

6 to 8 ounces (170 to 225 g) coconut kefir or coconut kombucha (purchased at health food store or www.bodyecology.com)

Pinch Celtic sea salt or pinch whole-plant ground stevia, optional

Squeeze the lime juice into the coconut liquid. Add salt or stevia, if using.

Yield: 3 to 4 one- to two-ounce (28 to 60 ml) beverages for baby

6

Think Outside the Box of Mac 'n' Cheese

Convenience Foods Can Cost You Your Child's Health

18 to 24 Months

Between 18 and 24 months, most toddlers will string a few words together into phrases. Your child might now be able to express what he would like to eat. Also, toddlers are realizing their independence and need to have a sense that they are in control, even if it means simply being able to pick the yellow cup over the blue cup or the apple over the banana.

If you have provided only PURE and Super POWER foods, you can easily trust that his body knows what it needs and allow him to choose.

As we'll discuss, the foods you choose to feed your child at this age will impact health on many levels—not only physical, but mental and emotional as well. Providing adequate ingredients from nutrient-worthy foods, while avoiding antinutrients (like those discussed in chapter 5), is the "recipe" for a healthy, happy child! This fourth pillar (nutrient-worth) of Super Nutrition will help steer your child through his next exciting milestones.

Dietary Influences on Tantrums and the Terrible Twos

Tantrums and problematic "terrible twos" behavior are expected and even somewhat accepted in childhood. Even in older children, behavioral issues, attention, mood, and learning problems are also starting to seem quite normal simply because they are so common. However, as we'll explain, diet can impact how children act, their attention spans, their ability to follow directions, and how they manage their emotions. How much of children's "bad" behavior today is due to "bad" diet? Too much!

Diet can either contribute to mood and behavioral problems or it can ameliorate—or even prevent—them, depending on which foods make up the diet. The quintessential toddler daily menu includes a breakfast of cereal or snack bars and juice or milk; a lunch of a white bread sandwich with jelly and sweetened peanut butter or a prepackaged meal, cookie, and juice box; snacks consist of cheesy grain-based crackers, chips, or "fruit" chews; and a dinner of pizza or pasta, accompanied by either juice or chocolate milk, and lastly dessert. As we'll explain in this chapter, this is a veritable diet of drinks and drugs! As such, behavior, mood, attention and physical health are all negatively impacted.

Drunken/Drugged Dietary Constituent	What It Creates	Drug(s) the Effects Mimic
Poorly digested grains	dietary opiates, excitotoxins, and endocannabinoids	morphine, heroine, and marijuana
Poorly digested pasteurized milk	dietary opiates, excitotoxins, and endocannabinoids	morphine, heroine, and marijuana
Sugar	dopamine	cocaine
Sugar	endorphins	morphine, opium, and heroine
Sugar	feeds yeast (by-products are ethanol and acetylaldehyde)	brain inebriation like alcoholic beverages
Sugar	adrenaline and norephinephrine	methamphetamine
Artificial sweeteners (aspartame), Flavor enhancers (MSG, hydrolyzed vegetable protein), Preservatives (carrageenan)	GABA, glutamate	marijuana

Some people are more "sensitive" or react more (*physically* and *emotionally*) to sugar, just as some adults develop alcoholism and others don't. Rather than being hardwired problems or just part of your child's personality, many of these mood and behavioral issues might actually stem from excessive sugar and sugar-sensitive responses. As reported in the *Journal of Attention Disorders*, sugar (and other processed foods) have direct effects on children's mental health.

But sugar is not the only culprit; other components of typical toddler diets also lead to behavior and mood problems. In fact, who would ever guess that toddlers are being fed a "drinks and drugs" diet that has effects similar to combining cocaine, vodka, beer, heroin, morphine, marijuana, and amphetamines? (See table, pg 144)

We urge you to *just say no* to the drunken and drugged diet of typical toddlers.

Hooked on bad-behavior foods. Due to these alcohol- and druglike effects on the body, the foods in typical toddler diets are actually habit forming; kids become biochemically dependent on their druglike foods. You might not realize that this is partly why your toddler vies (and cries) for sugary, flour-based foods. By giving in to these pleas, though, you act as an enabler, unknowingly feeding the habit with candy, pretzels, bagels, juice, cookies, and other treats.

Additives make for a troubled childhood. Further sapping the nutrient quality of foods are the unnatural ingredients used to extend shelf life, affect "mouthfeel," make fake food's color or flavor more appealing, etc. Moreover, the chemical additives in processed foods have been shown to lead to hyperactivity and impact mood in your child. And the converse is also true—by removing additives, you can help your child to be calm, content, and able to concentrate rather than irritable, distracted, and hyperactive.

Poor diet leads to disorder diagnoses. Too much sugar and the additives in typical toddler foods can significantly alter normal moods and behavior, leading to diagnoses of conditions such as attention deficit disorder, obsessive-compulsive disorder, learning disabilities, anger issues, and even depression. In children, more often than not, the set of symptoms leading to such diagnoses is likely related to a diet of drinks and drugs. For this reason, many experts now suggest a trial of dietary intervention before turning to prescription drugs for treatment.

The Typical Toddler Diet

It is normal to see toddlers eating diets predominantly of highly processed "kid foods," including prepackaged meals, macaroni and cheese, microwavable dinners, fast food, and even soda pop. Half of all meals are eaten away from home, and children's consumption of restaurant and fast-food meals rose by 300 percent between the 1970s and the 1990s.

Generally, most toddlers are subsisting on CRAP foods. But even those parents who focus on healthier fare can still end up with undernourished children. "Health" foods (like "kid" yogurt, whole-grain cereal, tofu, rice milk, probiotic-enriched juice, organic cereal bars, and low fat foods) are often just CRAP food in disguise and can lead to severe nutrient deficiencies and health problems. Most often they are not nutrient-worthy foods for growing children, and they can contain sugars, denatured proteins, and damaged, inflammatory vegetable oils.

Many of the foods in toddlers' diets (such as whole grain and soy products) contain naturally occurring "antinutrients," which block digestion as well as the absorption, conversion, and utilization of vitamins, minerals, enzymes, and hormones. Such foods can actually lead to severe nutrient *deficiencies*. They can also irritate the intestines, leading to tummy trouble like diarrhea, irritable bowel syndrome, gas/flatulence, bloating, and constipation.

A BETTER WAY TO NOURISH YOUR TODDLER

A child reared on processed, sugary, refined-grain foods will become programmed to seek out and subsist on anything *but* healthy foods throughout her life. By avoiding processed foods in your child's diet, for as long as you can, you will maintain your child's preferences for nutritious foods, creating a lifetime of good habits. Following are some other ways to protect your child's nutrition.

Don't switch to skim for the sake of low fat. While the AAP and USDA dietary guidelines recommend switching from whole milk to low-fat at 2 years old, this hallmark move to a "low-fat" diet for American children will deprive your child of important fat-soluble activators in their natural form, as well as important *protective* constituents. Studies have shown that *fat,* particularly in milk, is protective against rickets, osteoporosis, other mineral-deficiency diseases, arthritis, joint pain, calcification of arteries, cancer, heart disease, and diabetes. (See "A Low-Fat, Grown-Up Diet Is Not Best for Kids," page 148.)

Do fats right. The easiest way to get the right fats, in the correct amounts and ratios, in your toddler's diet is to let Nature take care of it for you. Use animal-based foods that have been pasture raised because their fats will be appropriately proportioned. When using plant fats, choose coconut and red-palm oil as well as some cold-pressed olive oil and avocado oil. Occasional use of unrefined nut and seed oils, such as walnut and sesame seed oils, as well as some use of flaxseed oil, is fine. Limiting processed foods will minimize exposure to unhealthy vegetable oils.

Create carb safety by knocking out antinutrients. Historically, traditional cultures purposefully *prepared* grains, nuts, beans, and seeds before consuming them, spending significant time to soak, ferment, sprout, and leaven these foods. By doing so, they improved digestion and gut health; reduced gas, cramps, and intestinal irritation; and ultimately improved overall energy and decreased allergies

Whole Grain Preparation

Specially prepared grains that are gluten free can occasionally be given to your child between 18 and 21 months of age and more commonly after 2 years. The methods used to prepare the grains make them the most nutritious and digestible.

Soaking: This simple process involves soaking grains (and beans) in enough water to cover with 2 tablespoons (28 g or 28 ml) of something acidic—plain yogurt, kefir, vinegar, or lemon juice—overnight (or about 7 to 24 hours). The soaking liquid should then be discarded, in most cases. Soaking allows ubiquitous lactobacilli and enzymes to neutralize antinutrients like phytic acid. Traditional peoples would also use soured raw milk for soaking.

Fermenting: This method involves the use of beneficial yeasts and bacteria to predigest starches and sugars in food, producing greater enzyme activity, more beneficial bacteria, lactic acid, vitamin K2, and an easier-to-digest food. The most commonly recognized example of fermented grains is sourdough bread.

Sprouting or germinating: Seeds (including grains, which are seeds) are sprouted or germinated using a moist, warm environment over a few days, allowing the seed to "believe" all conditions have been met to finally grow. When this occurs, their natural defense mechanisms dissipate—antinutrients, digestive blockers, and irritants are neutralized; enzyme content and nutrient content both increase, as well. Sprouts coming out of the seed can often be clearly seen.

Leavening: Natural leavening, or slow rising, is an ancient custom using fermenting "starters." This time-tested custom was lost with the advent of commercial yeast leaveners. Natural leavening also serves to neutralize harmful antinutrients in grains.

and diseases. We now know such traditional preparation enhances digestibility by *neutralizing antinutrients* and *increasing enzyme activity*. It also increases nutrition worth by *increasing beneficial bacteria, nutrient content, and availability*.

At this age, your baby's digestive system can handle some grains, but making those grains (as well as seeds, beans, and nuts) the most nutritious and least irritating and inflammatory requires special, traditional preparation (see sidebar and recipes in this chapter).

First, focus on whole grains. Whole grains from nature come with a "whole" package of nutrients and thus are far less disruptive to the body than refined grains. Then consider variety. Our society relies heavily on wheat and corn as our staple grains, and both are highly allergenic, especially when eaten frequently. Many other grains such as amaranth, quinoa, teff, millet, sorghum, and buckwheat (a fruit) provide an array of nutrients, don't contain gluten, and can be less irritating to the gut.

Instead of basing meals on grains (e.g., cereal or bagels, what kind of sandwich you'll have, what you'll serve over pasta), make grains a garnish or small side dish. The healthiest meals are based on protein, fats, vegetables, and greens—with fruit and nuts as dessert.

A Low-Fat, Grown-Up Diet Is Not Best for Kids

At your child's 2-year checkup, his doctor may suggest switching him to a low-fat diet, stressing the importance of grains, fruits, and vegetables while avoiding animal fats. Avoiding animal fats and animal proteins means that vegetable oils will be the predominant fats in your toddler's new low-fat, grown-up diet. But plant-based oils such as vegetable (soy), sunflower, corn, cottonseed, and canola are not traditional fats and are therefore "new" to the human body. Because they aren't animal based, they lack cholesterol, which, as we discussed in chapter 4, is critical for your toddler's brain development and gut health, and they lack nutrients and specific fatty acids found uniquely in animal fats.

Additionally, too many vegetable oils can cause organs and systems to flounder. They cause inflammation and internal body "rusting" and aging. These vegetable oils are predominantly polyunsaturated fats and are mostly made up of inflammatory omega-6 fatty acids. Since we all need a healthy balance between omega-3s and omega-6s, focusing primarily on vegetable oils means your toddler's fat ratio will be out of balance. This imbalance can disrupt cellular communication and can result in neurologic and psychological issues—aka: big-time health problems. To sum up, Williams Sears, M.D., and Martha Sears, R.N, succinctly state in *The NDD*™ (Nutrient Defect Disorder) *Book*, "the *healthier the fats, the healthier the cell membrane, the healthier the child.*" Your child also gets these inflammatory fats if he's consuming factory-farmed meats since the "grains" fed to farm animals are soy and corn (which are rich in unhealthy omega-6s); while fat from pastured (grass-fed) animals and wild-caught fish are higher in omega-3s.

Not all omega-6s are bad for you, though; *some* have health benefits. Chickpeas, nuts, borage oil, black currant seed, mom's milk, and evening primrose oil are sources the particular omega-6s fatty acids that are healthy.

Experts, like Dr. Sears and Judy Converse (*Special-Needs Kids Eat Right*), R.D., each warn that too many vegetable oils the following (the unhealthy omega-6s) can lead to or be associated with:

▸ Poor school performance

▸ Problems in autistic and ADHD children

▸ Misbehaviors: impulsive, aggressive, and angry

▸ Mood swings: sad, angry outbursts; anxious; and aggression

- Dyspraxia (poor gross motor coordination)
- Vision problems: decreasing acuity, dry eyes
- Skin: dry, flaky, scaly "chicken skin"
- Allergies: asthma, hay fever
- "-itis" illnesses: dermatitis, bronchitis, colitis, and arthritis
- Dyslexia
- Poor learning (in animal studies)

Trans fats. Hydrogenation is the process that transforms liquid oils into solids at room temperature (think shortening or margarine). When hydrogenated, vegetable oils become trans fats. Trans fats are the most unhealthy fats, having had their very molecular structure manipulated. They increase risk for cardiovascular disease, diabetes, and cancer; they cause inflammation and lead to obesity, infection, and illness. Further, trans fats eaten by mom lower her baby's birth weight and reduce the quality of her milk.

What They Don't Tell You about GMOs

GMOs (genetically modified organisms) look just like their natural counterparts and even taste like them, but their DNA is nothing like what Mother Nature made. Biotech companies use bacteria and viruses to force DNA from other sources into recipient DNA. They "engineer" seeds to produce their own insecticides or to be able to survive being sprayed with massive quantities of pesticides. Appallingly, GMO corn (designed to contain its own insecticide) is regulated by the Environmental Protection Agency because it is actually classified as an insecticide.

While most industrialized countries are either against GMO foods or require them to be labeled, the United States takes an innocent-until-proven-guilty stance, so no tests are required that *prove* they are safe. Lab animals, though, show early signs of cancer when fed GMO foods, and those working in the fields experience high rates of asthma, allergies, and skin rashes. Consuming GMO means you're getting more toxic exposure from pesticides since those crops are sprayed much more. Workers who apply pesticides have had severe allergic reactions to GMO plants. Further, mutated genes in GMO crops have been shown to spread to human cells when eaten and are implicated in increased immune reactions (similar to those seen in allergies and infections).

"GMO" COULD STAND FOR GENETICALLY MODIFIED OIL

Today's popular vegetable oils are also mostly made from genetically modified organisms (GMOs), which is yet another reason to avoid them. Canola, soy, corn, and cottonseed oils are almost always genetically modified. (And note that oils labeled simply "vegetable" are soy. (For more information on soy, see Chapter 8.) While Americans are not well educated on the dangers or risks of consuming GMO foods, European Union countries, Japan, New Zealand, Korea, Australia, and China all have either demanded GMO labeling or banned GMOs (like Austria, Hungary, and Peru).

While no large-scale studies have been funded, genetically modified foods have the potential for putting your child at greater risk for developing allergies and having other immune-related issues. There are also likely effects from incorporating the unnatural DNA in GMO foods into our bodies, such as increasing antibiotic resistance, organ abnormalities, future fertility problems, and cancer. With 70 percent of our foods containing GMOs, and no labeling required in the United States, we're taking grave risks with the health of our children, as well as the future of all food.

The Toddler Tantrum Solution

When we consider the effects of typical toddler diets high in sugar, antinutrient-containing foods, chemicals, and GMOs, is it any wonder that kids have skyrocketing problems with learning, attention, anxiety, depression, sensory processing, aggression, emotion, and mood conditions? Not to mention other 3C conditions like obesity, metabolic syndrome, heart disease, and diabetes?

If you feed your toddler a diet focused on optimal nutrition, based on Super Nutrition guidelines, he is more likely to have a better disposition and less likely to have excessive mood swings and behavioral outbursts.

TAKE THE SUGAR OUT, PUT THE PROTEIN AND FAT IN

In her book *Little Sugar Addicts: End the Mood Swings, Meltdowns, Tantrums, and Low Self-Esteem in Your Child Today*, Kathleen DesMaisons, Ph.D., pioneer and expert in the field of addictive nutrition, shares the straightforward relationship: Food affects feelings and feelings affect behavior. She writes, "Changing your child's food can give you back his sweet and loving side." Avoiding refined flour and sweeteners, while also regularly including protein with vegetables (avoiding all-carb meals or snacks), "can help . . . [children] focus, contribute to weight loss, alter blood sugar levels, eliminate mood swings, and defuse rage." Defusing rage is particularly important in young toddlers who can't express emotion well, which leads to tantrums.

CONTROL MOODS WITH REGULAR MEALS AND MINI-MEALS

Going *too* long without food can negatively impact hormones and brain chemicals. Dr. DesMaisons warns in *Little Sugar Addicts*: "Junk foods, soda . . . and *missed meals* activate the worst of what sugar sensitivity sets up." The drop in blood sugar resulting from a missed meal or snack can lead to a meltdown.

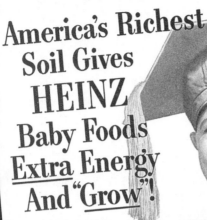

America's Richest Soil Gives HEINZ Baby Foods Extra Energy And "Grow"!

• • YOUR BABY'S HEALTH AND GROWTH demand the mineral-rich, vitamin-packed fruits and vegetables produced on America's most fertile farmlands! That's why Heinz locates its modern baby food kitchens right in the heart of these superior growing regions!

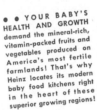

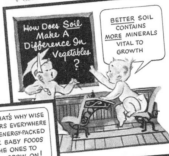

How Does Soil Make A Difference On Vegetables?

BETTER SOIL CONTAINS MORE MINERALS VITAL TO GROWTH

RIGHT! THAT'S WHY HEINZ BABY FOODS ARE GROWN IN THE NATION'S GARDEN SPOTS!

AND THAT'S WHY WISE MOTHERS EVERYWHERE MAKE ENERGY-PACKED HEINZ BABY FOODS THE ONES TO GROW ON!

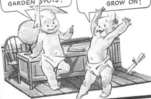

Doctors everywhere recommend Heinz Baby Foods because—

1 Heinz fruits and vegetables are raised in the nation's most fertile soil!

2 Heinz kitchens are located in the heart of these regions —to save time between field and kettle!

3 Heinz Baby Foods are scientifically cooked for higher nutritive value — *finer flavor, color and texture!*

4 Heinz quality is controlled by laboratory methods to assure uniformity.

5 Heinz quality is maintained at your grocer's. Heinz salesmen check supplies for *freshness!*

6 You know these baby foods taste good because they're *Heinz*—with an 82-year quality reputation.

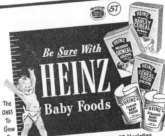

Be Sure With HEINZ Baby Foods

The ONES To Grow On

Complete Line Includes Over 50 Varieties
Strained Foods • Junior Foods • Pre-Cooked Cereal Food
Pre-Cooked Barley Cereal • Pre-Cooked Oatmeal

111

Though it's best to avoid constant grazing, children are in need of more frequent meals and snack intervals than adults are (children are typically hungry every 3 hours or so). According to Elizabeth Lipski, Ph.D., in *Digestive Wellness*, "Small, frequent meals keep children's energy levels even and their minds alert. Snacking reduces the incidence of children's tantrums."

However, snacking does not mean giving your child treats and processed foods. Better than thinking of them as snacks—too often associated with "treats"—think of them as "mini-meals," composed of animal protein, animal fat, and natural carbohydrates. Mini-meals are often parents' biggest challenge, as generally, the go-to snacks are refined flour based—and sugar filled. Instead, try those listed below:

▸ Beef snack sticks, pemmican (a meat-based "power bar"), pepperoni, and more from www.uswellnessmeats.com
▸ Presoaked homemade nut butter with apples or celery
▸ Raw cheese chunks
▸ Raw cottage cheese and diced fruit or peas and diced chicken
▸ Deviled eggs and olives
▸ Apple, walnut, chicken, and avocado salad

Decay and the Dentist

At 2 years old, it is time for your baby's first trip to the dentist. Although cavities and fillings are a very common part of childhood, humans are the only species with such rates of dental decay. Nearly half of all kids ages 2 to 11 have had cavities, and recent research indicates these rates are *increasing*.

Diet is a large part of what causes tooth decay, and the dietary element that is worst for teeth is, of course, sugar. Studies from the *Journal of Dental Research* show that sugar particularly *feeds* cavity-causing bacteria and pulls nutrients *away* from the outer portions of the teeth, making them malnourished and weak. Further, animals fed low-sugar diets have less plaque on their teeth. Researchers conclude that sugar clearly promotes cavities.

TODAY'S TEETH STARVE FOR MINERALS

Children's diets are significantly lacking in minerals, which historically have been richly found in foods. But modern foods are mineral poor because the soil from which they grow has become nutrient depleted. Compared to nutrient values in food five decades ago, broccoli now has half the calcium, cauliflower has 60 percent of the vitamin C, and watercress only 12 percent of the iron. Without these minerals, our teeth and bones suffer, as do various organs and biochemical systems that also rely on minerals. The importance of minerals reaches beyond *dental* health, as teeth are "windows" to the rest of the body: When dental health deteriorates, so does overall health.

Of the few minerals children *do* get in their diets, many of them aren't usable. This is because minerals can only be used if "activated." They need specific fat-soluble vitamins to assist them. Vitamins, A, D3, and K2, found in pastured-animal foods and fats, seafood, and lacto-fermented food and drinks are the magic mineral activators.

A RECIPE FOR HEALTHY TEETH

Just as a diet based on Super Nutrition protects your child's *body*, so it does his *teeth*. Basing his diet on animal foods is wise. Studies in the *Journal of Dental Research* report that protein consumption does not lead to dental decay because it doesn't feed the bacteria that cause cavities (nor does it disrupt minerals), as refined carbohydrates do.

Notably, dietary fat seems to *protect* teeth! Researchers state that "most [diet and cavity] studies . . . indicate that the effect of [fats and] oils is to reduce cavities." This is likely because fats coat the teeth and prevent acid from eating away at enamel, while also facilitating tooth mineralization because the mineral-activators are fat-soluble, needing dietary fat to be effective.

According the National Institutes of Health, "Building your children's 'bone bank' account is a lot like saving for their education: The more they can put away when they're young, the longer it should last as they get older." Building strong teeth, bones, and bodies relies on minerals and their fat-soluble activators vitamins D3, A, and K2.

Regularly feeding your child foods rich in minerals and fat-soluble activators, while avoiding foods that deplete minerals and create imbalances (sugar, soy, unprepared whole grains, white flour, and vegetable fats), translates into a great investment in your baby's health account.

Mom to Mom / Always try new recipes twice. Sometimes the first time is just a trial run and the second time is a smashing success.

Recipes That Go Beyond Mac 'n' Cheese

Grain-based foods can expand the diet and menu for your toddler. The recipes we provide are healthy ways to incorporate these foods into your child's diet. We offer advice on how to prepare whole grains and whole-grain flours before using them in recipes, and these suggestions might—at first—seem daunting and too time consuming. This method of cooking does take some forethought, but know that you are providing the best, most digestible and nutrient-worthy foods for your growing toddler that won't have the harmful repercussions of "regular" whole grains or even worse: refined grains.

FEEDING AT 18 TO 21 MONTHS

Between 18 and 21 months, you can introduce gluten-free grains, raw greens, and higher-fiber raw vegetables. For a more complete list of acceptable foods at this age, see the Food Introduction Timeline on page 222.

Whole Grain Preparation

Whole grains can be prepared to be most nutritious and most digestible for your baby. Then they can either be used in their whole form or stored and ground (as needed) into recipes that call for flour.

Whole grains found in "kernel" form at health food stores include millet, teff, amaranth, and quinoa. These are the best grains—along with oatmeal, brown or wild rice, sorghum, and buckwheat—to feed to your child first because they are gluten-free; gluten is a very difficult protein to digest and as such is a digestive irritant and potential allergen. Since wheat, rye, and barley contain gluten, we recommend postponing their introduction until after 2 years of age or at least only given infrequently at this age.

For the Grains:

1 cup (about 80 g) whole grains

2 cups (475 ml) warm water

2 tablespoons (28 g plain yogurt, or (28 ml) lemon juice, raw vinegar, or whey (see Homemade Whey, page 64)

Combine the ingredients in a glass or ceramic bowl. Stir the mixture. Cover and leave at room temperature for 7 to 24 hours.

Either prepare immediately in whole form (see Notes) or drain and dry for later grinding into flour (directions below).

Notes
- Whole quinoa does well in beanless chili: Soak 1 cup (173 g) quinoa in 3 cups (700 ml) water with 1 tablespoon (15 g) yogurt, (15 ml) whey, kefir, vinegar, or lemon juice for 12 to 24 hours. Rinse and drain.

Mom to Mom / To make them more practical, we advise soaking whole grains and drying them (and then storing them) as a project for one weekend per month. When a recipe calls for flour, this pre-prepared whole grain can simply be ground in a coffee-bean grinder in a matter of seconds and ready for the recipe.

In 2 cups (475 ml) of Souper Stock (page 56; to further increase nutrient content), bring the quinoa to a boil and then simmer, covered, for an hour. Mix with ground beef, garlic, a pinch of chile pepper, and cooked onion and stewed tomatoes.
- Whole millet makes a nice casserole-style accompaniment to meat: After soaking (as described above), don't drain, but bring to boil; then cover tightly and simmer for 45 minutes. Add butter and salt to taste.

For the Flour:

Drain soaked grains and dry with a dehydrator or on paper towel-lined cookie sheets (changing the paper towel several times). You can also use the lowest setting in your oven or toaster oven (150°F [66°C] to 170°F [77°C]).

Store *completely* dried grains in a glass container in the refrigerator or cool pantry.

To make flour, grind the dried grains fresh in a coffee-bean grinder, grain mill, or Vitamix to yield the amount of flour you need for a recipe.

Store-Bought Flour Preparation

Flour that is freshly ground just before use in a recipe is ideal and ultimately most nutritious. Once grain is ground, it begins to oxidize and lose nutrients; therefore, flour from the grocery store, even if whole grain, is not as superior as freshly ground flour from grains prepared as above. In many cases, however, the convenience of purchasing already-ground whole-grain flour is necessary. You can and should prepare this flour to be more digestible and nutritious for your toddler.

Kamut, spelt, and whole-grain wheat flour can be used, but because they contain gluten, they are better postponed until 2 years of age. Gluten-free flours are best.

1¹/₃ cups (about 160 g) purchased whole-grain flour (millet, brown rice, sorghum, teff, coconut)

¹/₂ cup (120 ml) water or ¹/₂ cup (120 ml) raw milk or ¹/₂ cup (115 g) raw yogurt (if using yogurt, omit tablespoon below)

1 tablespoon (15 g) yogurt, or (15 ml) whey, vinegar, or lemon juice

Stir the ingredients together in a glass bowl. Leave to soak overnight, covered, at room temperature. Use in the morning or store in the refrigerator for use later that day or possibly the next.

Notes

- Use this "wet" flour, measure for measure, in recipes for crepes, pancakes, muffins, and more.
- You might need to reduce the liquid called for in your recipe, as the prepared-flour mixture will contain liquid.

Rice Preparation

Though rice is low in mineral-blocking phytic acid, it is still a grain and can be made more digestible and nutritious through sprouting or soaking or a lengthened cook time before eating. Organic whole-grain rice can be short, medium, or long grain and should be colorful (not white): black, wild, or brown. Tru Roots brand sells a pregerminated (sprouted) rice for commercial sale at health food stores.

1 cup (about 185 g) rice

2 cups (475 ml) water

1 tablespoon (15 ml) whey, vinegar, lemon juice, or (15 g) yogurt

Combine the ingredients in a glass or ceramic bowl. Stir the mixture. Cover and leave at room temperature overnight (at least 7 hours). Drain and rinse.

Cook rice as directed on the package, either using water or Souper Stock (page 56; reduced by ¹/₄ cup [60 ml]).

Alternate technique:

1 cup (about 185 g) rice

2 tablespoons (28 g) butter

2 cups (475 ml) Souper Stock (page 56)

In a skillet, sauté and continously stir the rice in the butter over medium-low heat. When the rice and liquid are cloudy, add the premade stock. Bring to a soft boil and simmer 10 to 12 minutes.

Reduce heat to low, cover, and allow to cook for about 2 hours.

Optional: Add 1 tablespoon (7 g) of Bernard Jensen's gelatin (www.radiantlifecatalog.com) to the stock.

Notes

- TruRoots brand is available at health food stores and is already germinated (sprouted). You can follow the package directions or grind into brown rice flour.

Bean Preparation

Beans, like grains, must be prepared to be digestible and nutritious. Here are rules of thumb for common kinds of beans, as provided by Wise Traditions in Food, Farming and the Healing Arts, *the quarterly magazine of the Weston A. Price Foundation, Winter http://www.westonaprice.org/ journal/1563.html, 2006.*

1 cup (about 250 g) beans

2 cups (475 ml) water

2 to 3 tablespoons (28 to 45 ml) whey, lemon juice, vinegar, or (28 to 45 g) yogurt

2 to 4 minced garlic cloves, optional

Soak as specified below, per type of bean. Rinse and drain. Cook in slow cooker for 4 to 8 hours; the beans will be ready to eat after 4 hours but can be cooked longer for easier digestion.

Optional: Add minced garlic to cooking beans.

Notes

- *Black beans,* soak for 18 to 24 hours; *lentils,* soak for 10 hours; *fava beans,* soak for 10 hours (be sure to discard the liquid and remove the outer skin of the fava beans before using in a recipe); *dried and split peas,* best soaked for 10 hours in filtered water with a pinch of baking soda; *brown, white, and kidney beans,* soak for 18 to 24 hours in filtered water.

Sprouting Grains and Beans

In addition to the soaking method of preparation, grains and beans can be sprouted. Sprouts can be used in salads, sandwiches, porridges, casseroles, and more.

Revisit the nut and seed sprouting directions on page 136, following these guidelines: *Wheat, rye, and barley,* rinse 2 to 3 times per day for 3 to 4 days; *buckwheat,* rinse 2 to 3 times per day for 2 days; *kidney, lima, and black beans,* rinse 3 to 4 times per day for 3 days; *lentils,* rinse 3 times per day for 2 to 3 days.

Most grains and beans will develop tiny sprouts when germination has been successful. When sprouted, store in the refrigerator.

Old-Fashioned Porridge

In the style of Goldilocks and the Three Bears, porridge is an excellent way to enjoy prepared grains, like oatmeal. In addition, buckwheat groats, whole teff, and amaranth are also good for breakfast porridge. Kamut, spelt, and ground rye can also be used, but since they contain gluten, they are better postponed until age 2. Because oats have enzymes to help with fat digestion, they go well with butter or cream. Combining fats with grains also improves nutrient absorption and helps maintain even blood sugar.

1 cup (about 80 g) grains

1 cup (235 ml) water

2 tablespoons (30 g) yogurt (or [28 ml] whey, see options, page 64)

Stir together the ingredients in a bowl. Allow to sit overnight, covered, at room temperature.

In the morning, bring 1 cup (235 ml) water to a boil and then add the grain mixture.

Stir and cook for 5 minutes or until thickened to porridge consistency.

Yield: 2 servings

Notes

- Serve with butter, fruit, and cinnamon or mix with yogurt and fruit.
- Old-fashioned, slow-cook, rolled, steel-cut, or cracked oats are best; instant or quick-cooking oats are not recommended.
- If using buckwheat, toast the groats before soaking for less stickiness.
- As an alternate technique, soak 1 cup (about 80 g) grains in 1 cup (235 ml) warm water with the juice of half a lemon overnight. Drain and rinse in the morning. Add 1 to 2 cups (235 to 475 ml) water and a pinch of Celtic sea salt. This cooks up quickly—in about 5 minutes.

Flying Saucer Pizzas

These fun mini pizzas are easy and yummy. Let your little one top his own pizza or arrange the toppings into a smiley face or flower. This recipe uses ground prepared whole grains to make the flour.

1¼ cups (about 150 g) flour (preferably presoaked, dried, and freshly ground)

¼ cup (32 g) arrowroot starch

2 tablespoons (28 g) softened organic butter, plus more for greasing pizza pan

½ teaspoon salt, plus more

1 egg

½ cup (120 ml) liquid (raw milk, yogurt, homemade coconut milk [page 93])

2 teaspoons basil

2 teaspoons oregano

Egg white, lightly beaten, optional

¾ cup (184 g) tomato sauce (homemade or store bought, sugar free—can also be infused with Souper Stock [page 56])

1 cup (about 150 g) grated pizza cheese (preferably raw)

Toppings like tomato slices or farm-fresh pepperoni, optional

Preheat the oven to 350°F (180°C, gas mark 4). Mix the flour and starch with the butter. Add the salt, egg, liquid, and spices. Stir until mixed.

Grease a 12-inch (30 cm) pizza round or cookie sheet with butter. Pour the dough on the sheet and spread over the surface. Brush with egg white and sprinkle with sea salt (optional). Top the pizzas with the tomato sauce. Cover with cheese and add optional toppings. Bake for 10 to 12 minutes until cheese is melted and golden.

Yield: 1 round or 1 "square" pizza

Notes

- If using purchased whole-grain flour, prepare it the night before by soaking 2/3 cup (80 g) flour with 1 tablespoon (15 g) yogurt and 1/4 cup (60 ml) water overnight, covered; then proceed with the recipe.
- *Variation*: Instead of "dough," use portobello mushrooms.

Blueberry Breakfast Crepes with Raspberry Syrup

Crepes are French in origin and are basically a thin pancake. These crepes do not use the typical white flour that spikes blood sugar without offering much nutrition. The syrup recipe is adapted from Nourishing Traditions *by Sally Fallon and uses only natural sweeteners with some nutritive value. It's far better than the corn syrup–based stuff at the grocery store.*

For the Crepes:

4 eggs

1/2 teaspoon vanilla extract

1/2 teaspoon ground cinnamon

1 small brown-spotted banana, mashed, or 1/2 cup (125 g) Apple Spread (page 161)

1/4 cup (20 g) shredded coconut

1/4 cup (32 g) arrowroot starch

3 tablespoons (42 g) butter or ghee

1/2 cup (75 g) blueberries, rinsed and picked over

Mix the eggs, vanilla, cinnamon, banana or apple spread, coconut, and arrowroot until a batter forms.

In a small nonstick skillet or crepe pan, warm the butter or ghee over medium-low heat until it is almost brown. Pour about 1/4 cup (55 g) of the mixture into the pan and tilt the pan to coat the bottom surface. Sprinkle some blueberries over the batter.

Flip the crepe when the edges easily lift, about 1 to 2 minutes. Cook 1 minute on the other side.

For the Raspberry Syrup (make ahead of time):

4 cups (500 g) raspberries, washed and well mashed, pressed down into a quart-size mason jar

2 teaspoons Celtic sea salt

¼ cup (48 g) Rapunzel brand Rapadura or other whole-foods sweetener

¼ cup (60 ml) whey (see Homemade Whey, page 64)

Mix the salt, Rapadura, and whey and pour into the jar. Mix thoroughly.

Add filtered water just to the top of the berries, leaving at least 1 inch (2.5 cm) to the top of the jar.

Cover tightly and allow to sit at room temperature for 2 days.

Yield: 4 to 6 crepes

Note

- Store in the refrigerator and use syrup within 8 weeks.

What to Watch For at the Grocery Store

If you do purchase packaged foods, strive to avoid the following worst ingredients:

- Hydrogenated or partially hydrogenated oils, trans fats
- High fructose corn syrup, corn syrup, "corn sugar" (another name for HFCS)
- Aspartame
- Sucralose
- Saccharin
- MSG
- Propyl gallate
- Hydrolyzed vegetable protein
- Dyes (red 3, yellow 6, blue 1, blue 2, green 3)
- Acesulfame potassium (or acesulfame K)
- Butylated hydroxyanisole (BHA)
- Brominated flour
- Potassium bromate
- Sodium benzoate
- Sodium nitrite

Raw Veggies, Salad, and Dressing

At this age, tender greens (like butterleaf), carrots, cucumbers, bell peppers, and tomatoes are low enough in fiber to be enjoyed raw. These foods have great nutrient worth, as they are bright and colorful—indicative of their nutritional value. Try offering this to your child as his first salad! Make a "ranch" dressing with whole-milk yogurt, mixed herbs and spices, and sea salt; or an "Italian" version with 2 parts olive, avocado, walnut, or sesame oil to 1 part raw apple cider or raw coconut vinegar; add seasonings to taste.

Sprouted-Corn Quesadillas with Homemade Salsa

Corn is a grain and should be sprouted and soaked with lime water, as "masa" flour is—a process which makes vitamin B3 available, enhancing the nutrient quality of the corn. Use health food store (non-GMO) sprouted-corn tortillas as a convenient way to healthfully consume corn in a more digestible and less nutrient-blocking form. The salsa is adapted from Nourishing Traditions *by Sally Fallon and is a delicious way to incorporate a lacto-fermented food. Make it 2 days before you plan to have quesadillas.*

Warm butter or another fat in a skillet. Place sprouted tortillas with grated fresh cheese and meat of choice (leftover chicken, salmon, or organic, nitrite/nitrate-free lunch meat). Fold and flip. Cut into triangle wedges or smaller bites, as your child needs.

Lacto-Fermented Salsa:

4 tomatoes

2 small, finely chopped onions

3/4 cup (108 g) chile peppers

6 to 8 cloves minced garlic

1 bunch chopped cilantro

1 teaspoon dried oregano

Juice of 2 lemons

1 tablespoon (15 g) Celtic sea salt

4 tablespoons (60 ml) whey (or additional tablespoon salt)

1/4 cup (60 ml) filtered water

Bring a small pot of water to a boil. Set aside a separate bowl filled with ice water.

Meanwhile, cut a small X in the bottom of each tomato and remove the stem scar from the top. Boil each tomato, one at a time, for 5 to 15 seconds and then plunge into ice water. Peel, deseed, and dice each one.

Mix the remaining ingredients with the tomatoes and press down well in a mason jar. Add water if necessary to just cover the tamped-down mixture, leaving at least 1 inch (2.5 cm) to the top of the jar.

Cover and leave for 48 hours at room temperature and then store in refrigerator.

Yield: 1 quart (950 ml)

Apple or Pear Spread

This spread can be used in place of jelly or can be used as "applesauce" for an accompaniment to lunch or a delicious treat after dinner. Whereas commercial jams and jellies (and often even homemade) are loaded with nutrient-zapping sugar, this alternative is tasty and nutritious, particularly if lacto-fermented with whey.

3 tablespoons (42 g) butter or (51 g) coconut oil

5 apples or pears, core and sliced.

2 tablespoons (14 g) ground cinnamon

1 tablespoon (15 ml) vanilla extract for apples or 2 teaspoons almond extract for pears

2 teaspoons Celtic sea salt, divided

2 tablespoons (28 ml) whey, divided (see Homemade Whey, page 64)

Warm the coconut oil or butter in a skillet over medium-low heat. Add the apples or pears, cinnamon, and vanilla or almond extract. Stir to coat the fruit.

Cook, covered, until the fruit is soft.

Remove from heat and purée with a blender. (Take caution when puréeing hot foods.)

Distribute the purée evenly between 2 Mason jars, and add the salt and whey to each jar.

Cover tightly and allow to stand at room temperature for 24 hours.

Notes

- Don't peel the fruit, as the peel retains important nutrients.
- This may be stored in the refrigerator for about 4 weeks.

Cod Liver Oil

At this age, your child has higher requirements for the nutrients in cod liver oil. Up his dosage to $1\frac{1}{2}$ teaspoons of high-quality cod liver oil (or $\frac{3}{4}$ teaspoon fermented). At this dose, your child should be getting sufficient vitamin D, so no additional D is needed.

"Yorkshire" Marrow Custard

This is a gluten free, nutrient-rich variation of Yorkshire pudding, which is a traditional English recipe made with eggs, flour, and roast beef drippings. The recipe is adapted from "Bone Marrow Custard" by Sally Fallon Morell in her Growing Healthy Children *presentation.*

2 pounds (910 g) marrow bones

1 cup (235 ml) farm-fresh or non-ultrapasteurized heavy cream

2 egg yolks

1 whole egg

Celtic sea salt and pepper to taste

Preheat the oven to 300°F (150°C, gas mark 2).

Simmer marrow bones in water and extract 2 ounces (55 g) softened marrow. Blend the marrow with cream and eggs and season to taste. Pour into 4 buttered ramekins (or lined muffin tins). Bake at for about 20 minutes or until the custards are set.

This is great to serve with meat dishes.

Yield: 4 servings

Grilled Cheese Sandwiches with "Cornmeal Spoon Bread"

Most breads, even if "whole grain," contain nutrient-depleting white flour, as well as one or more forms of sugar. This tasty bread, adapted from Nourishing Traditions *by Sally Fallon, can be sliced thin and used as sandwich bread for cold or toasted sandwiches.*

For Bread:

2 cups (240 g) masa flour (see note)

2 cups (475 ml) filtered water

2 cups (460 g) yogurt or kefir

Mix the ingredients in a bowl and let stand, covered, on your counter for 24 to 48 hours.

To Finish the Recipe:

1 onion, finely chopped

2 tablespoons (28 g) butter

5 eggs, separated

1 teaspoon Celtic sea salt

1/8 teaspoon cayenne pepper

2 teaspoons aluminum-free baking powder

Preheat the oven to 375°F (190°C, gas mark 5).

Sauté the onion in the butter. Blend the egg yolks into the prepared flour mixture. Add the salt, cayenne pepper, cooked onions, and baking powder. Stir until combined.

Beat the egg whites in a separate bowl until stiff; then fold into the yolk mixture.

Pour the mixture into a buttered 9 × 13-inch (23 × 33 cm) glass baking dish and bake for about 45 minutes until knife comes out clean from center.

For Sandwiches:

Baked bread can be sliced into "sandwich" bread once cooled. (Cut larger, "breadloaf-size" squares in the pan and cut each square horizontally to make two "slices.") Butter, sauté, and fill with leftover meat or organic, nitrite/nitrate-free lunch meat and slices of fresh cheese.

Optional: Enjoy this sandwich open faced with a fried egg on top, croque madame–style.

Note

- To make masa flour, non-GMO cornmeal must be soaked in lime water. Make lime water by placing 1 inch (2.5 cm) pickling lime into a 2-quart (1.9 L) jar filled with water. Shake well, cover, and let stand overnight. Sediment will settle at the bottom.

Carefully pour out 2 cups (475 ml) of lime water. Add 2 cups (244 g) of freshly ground cornmeal (or store-bought organic cornmeal) and soak for 7 hours.

FEEDING AT 21 TO 24 MONTHS

Between 21 and 24 months, you can introduce properly prepared gluten grains, properly prepared legumes, and shellfish. For a more complete list of acceptable foods at this age, see the Food Introduction Timeline on page 222.

Berry Jam

3 cups (about 435 g) fresh or frozen blueberries, blackberries, strawberries, halved, or (375 g) raspberries

2 tablespoons (40 g) maple syrup

3 to 4 tablespoons (21 to 28 g) Bernard Jensen's gelatin (www.radiantlifecatalog.com)

In a pan on over medium-low heat, simmer the berries. Stir occasionally and mash the fruit. Add the syrup and gelatin, stirring in very slowly to fully dissolve the gelatin.

Remove from the heat and purée with a hand blender or regular blender. (Have caution when puréeing hot mixtures.)

Let cool on the counter and then store in a mason jar in the refrigerator.

Yield: About 2 to 3 cups (640 to 960 g)

Note: This "jam" will liquefy when exposed to warm temperatures for any duration.

Cottage Cheese

If you can find fresh, raw cottage cheese from your local dairy, it is a great treat. Mix with chives or try fruit and sprinkle with cinnamon; or mix with green peas and diced chicken.

Cholent (Traditional Baked Beans)

A traditional Jewish food, cholent is a slow-cooked dish—making beans both digestible and delicious. This recipe is adapted from Wise Traditions in Food, Farming and the Healing Arts, *the quarterly magazine of the Weston A. Price Foundation, Winter http://www.westonaprice.org/journal/1563.html, 2006.*

The Night Before:

¾ cup (138 g) barley or buckwheat

2 tablespoons (28 ml) lemon juice, whey, vinegar, or (30 g) yogurt (see Homemade Whey, page 64

1¼ cups (about 269 g) brown or white beans

Soak the barley or buckwheat overnight in water with lemon juice, whey, vinegar, or yogurt.

Separately, rinse the beans and place in a pot with 6 cups (1.4 L) simmering water and soak for 18 to 24 hours (if possible, drain and add fresh, simmering water a few times during this time).

To Finish the Recipe:

2 tablespoons (28 ml) olive oil, or use (28 g) butter

1 large onion, coarsely chopped

3 to 6 cloves garlic, minced

1 pound (455 g) beef brisket

1 smoked beef bone or marrow bone

1½ pounds (340 g) potatoes (like Yukon gold), cut into chunks

1½ tablespoons (11 g) Hungarian paprika

1½ teaspoons Celtic sea salt and pepper

6 eggs

Preheat the oven to 200°F (93°C).

Heat the olive oil or butter in a skillet over medium-high heat and sauté the onion until golden. Remove from the heat.

Combine the drained barley, drained beans, cooked onion, garlic, brisket, bone, potatoes, and seasonings in a large baking dish or Dutch oven with a tightly fitting lid.

"Bury" the uncooked eggs in their shells beneath the mixture and add enough water to cover the mixture. Bake, tightly covered, for 12 to 18 hours.

When ready to serve, remove and shell the eggs and remove and slice the brisket. Serve them with the cholent.

Note

• This dish is best served with unpasteurized sauerkraut, pickles, or other lacto-fermented condiment.

Shellfish

Like fish, shellfish can be contaminated with pollutants. However, since shellfish (like other seafood) offer a unique and hardy blend of minerals, vitamins, and fat-soluble activators (vitamins A, D3, and K2), their benefits outweigh the risks. That said, we recommend your child consumes shellfish no more than 1 to 2 times per month. Shellfish, along with seaweed, is an excellent source of the very important mineral iodine. Alternatively, organic dulse flakes, a seaweed, can be found at your health food store and easily added to many dishes.

• *Scallops:* Sear in bacon fat or coconut oil.
• *Garlic Buttered Shrimp:* Warm butter and minced garlic and cook shrimp until lightly golden.
• *Coconut Shrimp:* Dip shrimp in beaten egg and then dip in shredded coconut. Sauté in preheated butter or coconut oil.
• *Oysters Rockefeller:* Purchase oysters on the half shell and cover with a mixture of Creamed Spinach (page 130), crumbled bacon, and grated fresh cheese; bake 10 minutes at 450°F (230°C, gas mark 8).
• *Lobster and crab:* Serve with drawn butter.

Note

• Instead of coconut shrimp, you can substitute fish or chicken, in which case add a bit of arrowroot starch, coconut flour, and/or grated cheese to the "breading" mixture.

Tomato Marrow Soup

This tomato soup is superior to other versions, as it is infused with nutritious bone marrow. It is taken from the Weston A. Price Foundation website.

6 tomatoes

2 medium onions, sliced

3 tablespoons (42 g) butter or ghee

½ cup (120 ml) white wine or vermouth, optional

6 to 8 cups (1.4 to 1.9 L) beef Souper Stock (page 56)

4 ounces (115 g) bone marrow

Celtic sea salt, pepper, cayenne pepper to taste

Bring a small pot of water to a boil. Set aside a separate bowl filled with ice water.

Meanwhile, cut a small X in the bottom of each tomato and remove the stem scar from the top. Boil each tomato, one at a time, for 5 to 15 seconds, and then plunge into ice water. Peel, deseed, and chop each one.

Sauté the onions in the butter or ghee over medium-high heat until golden brown. Add the tomatoes, stirring until their liquid has evaporated. Add the white wine or vermouth, if using. Add the Souper Stock and bring to a simmer. Lower the heat to medium and simmer for 15 minutes, skimming off any froth that rises.

Remove from heat and add the bone marrow. Blend in a blender or in a Vitamix or regular blender. (Have caution when blending hot liquids.)

Yield: 8 servings

Note

- Serve with cultured cream, yogurt, sour cream, or coconut milk (make your own, page 93).

Homemade "Caroblettes"

Using naturally sweet carob means that no sweetener is needed to make these "chocolates." Since chocolate has caffeine, carob is better for toddlers.

1 cup (205 g) coconut oil

1 tablespoon (14 g) butter

¼ cup (65 g) natural peanut butter or nut butter (page 137) + 1 teaspoon butter

2 tablespoons (20 g) carob powder

¼ teaspoon Celtic sea salt

Melt and stir together the coconut oil, butter, and nut butter. Remove from the heat and stir in the carob and salt.

While warm, spoon into flexible molds or flexible ice-cube trays. Refrigerate until ready to eat.

Note

- Enjoy these just after removing from the refrigerator, as they will melt in your mouth and in your hands!

Carob Mousse Pops

These pops make for a yummy summer treat—and they're so much better for your child than the sugar-laden fudge pops offered from the ice-cream truck.

1²/₃ cups (395 ml) farm cream or non-ultrapasteurized heavy cream

³/₄ cup (175 ml) coconut milk or raw milk

3 tablespoons (30 g) carob powder

Mix ingredients together and spoon into ice-pop molds. Freeze until set.

Note

- You can use yogurt, coconut oil, coconut milk, or puréed avocado as a portion of the cream or in place of it.

Chicken Curry with Soaked Rice and Coconut "Chutney"

This is a fun, colorful, and palate-pleasing dish with a variety of flavors.

1 pound (455 g) chicken thighs or breasts

2 teaspoons ground curry

3 to 4 tablespoons (42 to 55 g) butter

Celtic sea salt, to taste

1 tablespoon (15 ml) fermented-soy, wheat-free tamari soy sauce, optional

1 cup (about 185 g) whole grain rice

1 cup (125 g) chopped apple

¹/₄ cup (35 g) unsulfured dried fruit, like raisins or dried mulberries

¹/₃ cup (28 g) shredded, unsweetened, unsulfured coconut

For the Chicken:

In a skillet, sauté the curry in butter to bring out the full flavor.

Add the chicken and add sea salt to taste. Season with fermented-soy, wheat-free tamari sauce (optional). Cook the chicken on both sides until the center is no longer pink. Mince or finely chop the chicken into bite-size chunks.

For the Rice:

Prepare your choice of rice as described on page 155.

For the "Chutney":

Mix together the fruit and coconut.

Top the minced chicken and rice with the chutney.

Pink Citrus Spritzer

Using the Pretty Pink Drink recipe on page 114, add the juice of half a lemon and a pinch of whole-plant stevia for a fun citrus-y beverage.

Macadamia Nut–Carob Coconut Balls

These easy treats can be brought to friends' birthday parties or celebrations.

Mix 1 cup (about 260 g) homemade macadamia nut butter (see recipe, page 137) or if necessary, use store bought

1 tablespoon (10 g) carob powder

½ cup (43 g) unsweetened, unsulfured, shredded coconut

In a medium bowl, combine the nut butter and carob powder and form into 1-inch (2.5 cm) balls. Roll in the coconut.

Yield: 6 to 8 balls

Recognize the Link between "Junk" Foods and Mental Health

A large 2011 study, published in PLoS One, of more than 3,000 eleven to eighteen year olds, demonstrated that adolescents who ate highly processed and junk-food diets were more prone to episodes of depression and anxiety. But by consuming more whole foods, the study showed that children had less depression and anxiety. A diet of whole foods, rather than one of highly-refined carbohydrate "junk" foods, serves the body—and the mind—well, as this study suggests. Notably, a more nutritious diet can actually reduce episodes of mental health problems! This demonstrates that diet directly impacts mood, perception, and attitude (and therefore emotions and behaviors)—for better or worse. Such findings have been shown in several studies on adults, but now it is quite clear that adolescents' mental health is equally impacted: negatively by poor diet or positively by a nutrient-rich diet. It is particularly poignant to note that 75 percent of psychiatric illnesses begin prior to adulthood; and once one has experienced depression, that person is likely to suffer with it again. Thus, by feeding your child well now (distinctly steering clear of highly-processed junk foods and focusing on nutrient-worthy whole foods), you are taking steps toward a better state of mental health throughout his entire life. For such reasons, we urge you to recognize this important connection between those treats, sweets, and convenience foods and your child's current and long-term moods, emotions, and overall mental health.

Fruit Cobbler

This lip-smacking cobbler is perfect for a second-birthday-party treat. The recipe is adapted from Nourishing Traditions *by Sally Fallon.*

8 peeled, cored, sliced apples; 8 ripe, sliced peaches; or 6 cups (870 g) blueberries

1 tablespoon (8 g) arrowroot starch

1/2 teaspoon ground cinnamon

Juice and grated rind of one lemon

2 tablespoons (24 g) Rapunzel brand Rapadura or other whole-foods sweetener

Preheat the oven to 350°F (180°C, gas mark 4).

Mix and gently toss the fruit with the arrowroot, cinnamon (omit if using blueberries), lemon juice and rind, and Rapadura. Place the mixture in a well-buttered glass baking dish.

For the Crumble:

3/4 cup (84 g) almond meal (ground from presoaked almonds; see page 137)

3/4 cup (96 g) arrowroot starch

6 tablespoons (85 g) softened butter

1/4 cup (48 g) Rapunzel brand Rapadura or other whole-foods sweetener

1/4 teaspoon Celtic sea salt

1 teaspoon vanilla extract

Mix all the crumble ingredients together. Top the fruit with the "crumble" mixture.

Bake for 1 hour. Serve warm with farm fresh cream that's been whipped until stiff.

Note

- Coconut palm sugar is also a sweetener option, though it does not retain as much nutrient value as Rapunzel Rapadura.

Mom's Diet Does Matter

Critical Feeding Information for Breast-Fed Babies

0 to 6 Months

If you've turned to this chapter first, congratulations on your commitment to provide the absolute best nourishment for your baby. This chapter contains critical information regarding nourishing your baby through nourishing yourself, both during pregnancy and while your child is breast-feeding. It focuses on you and *your diet* and how food choices can make you and your milk Super POWERful in supply and nutrition.

If you're reading this chapter after finishing chapter 6 (18 to 24 months), you might think this chapter isn't important if your baby is older than 6 months. Yet it is worthwhile, as it contains information regarding how to use Super Nutrition for yourself, as well as provides additional insights about infant nutrition. In this chapter, we provide more details on aspects of the Super Nutrition program, delicious recipes, and valuable information on supplements—for both you and your child.

The Magic of Mom's Milk

Infancy is a delicate and vulnerable time. After leaving the comfort of the womb, your baby's body undertakes many changes, from breathing air to swallowing milk. Her life lessons begin now, starting with mastering latching on to your nipple to learning how to get your attention. Her largest sense of comfort in this new world are the familiarities she brings from in utero: your heartbeat, breathing rhythm, and voice, all of which are combined when she's held and fed by you.

In the early 1900s, 95 percent of mothers nursed their babies. Today, according to the CDC, 75 percent of moms *try*, but only about 33 percent of babies are exclusively breast-fed for the first 3 months and only 13 percent are still being exclusively nursed at 6 months. At 1 year, only 2 percent are still getting some of mom's milk. These low breast-feeding statistics are surprising because countless international and national health authorities stress that "mom's" milk is the best source of nutrition for an infant for *at least* the first year of life and thus recommend breast-feeding *exclusively* (no water, juice, nonhuman milk, or foods) *for the first 6 months.*

Various studies and research tout the health benefits of breast-feeding for your baby, many of which you've likely already heard. Just a few of the benefits include improved speech and vision development, superior fine-motor coordination, and fewer behavioral problems; better bonding between mother and baby; higher IQ and better intellectual, cognitive, and neurodevelopment; fewer allergies and fewer ear, upper respiratory, and gastrointestinal infections; and less digestive distress and fewer food allergies.

Something you might *not* be aware of, however, is the awesome protective power of mom's milk. There is a 36 percent lower infant death rate in babies who were ever breast-fed. These babies are also offered protection from chronic childhood diseases and others such as multiple sclerosis, inflammatory bowel disease (like Crohn's and ulcerative colitis), arthritis, celiac disease, hypertension, high cholesterol, heart disease, type 1 diabetes, and obesity.

Human Milk—"Breast" Milk or "Mom's" Milk?

Though it is common to call human milk "breast" milk, we feel this unduly objectifies the breast and also incorrectly separates the milk from the mother. (We don't call bovine dairy "udder milk," do we?)

It is the *whole* mom (not just her breast) who is making milk for her baby—her nutrient stores, her diet, her energy, her hormones, her enzymes, and her time, effort, and enjoyment to nurse—so for this reason, we refer to human milk, more appropriately, as *mom's milk.*

Mom's Diet Matters

The most common advice given to nursing moms about nutrition is this: "Just don't drink, smoke, or do drugs. Keep taking your prenatal vitamin, and all will be fine." If more is said on the matter, it is usually only this: "Try to maintain a healthy diet, but if you have a few bad days, your body will take from you to give the baby what she needs."

Despite such lackadaisical advice around mom's diet during nursing, your diet is actually extremely important. What you eat and what you avoid both impact your baby's health. As Robert Sears, M.D., says in *Happy Baby: Organic Guide to the First 24 Months*, "when you're feeding Baby your breast milk, she *is* what *you* eat."

WHAT'S OKAY

While nursing, you can eat many of the things you were told to cut out while pregnant: sushi, soft and raw (unpasteurized) cheeses, pâté, deli meats, and raw eggs. If there is a family history of the 3C conditions in parents, siblings, or grandparents, it might be wise to avoid peanut butter (a legume, like soy); otherwise, natural, unsweetened peanut butter in limited quantities is fine. There is no reason to avoid seasonings, especially as your milk will change flavor with your diet—enriching your baby's palate. Raw honey, too, is fine for nursing moms (don't give raw honey to your baby, though, if under 1 year). Teas (white, green, black, and oolong) contain tannins, which are digestive irritants and can block protein digestion and mineral absorption (particularly iron), so should be used sparingly. Though herbal teas do not necessarily contain actual tea, but rather herbal infusions, we recommend talking to an herbalist to learn more about herbs while nursing.

WHAT'S NOT OKAY

There are some definite things to avoid while nursing to protect your baby. Smoking, "doing drugs," and drinking too much alcohol while nursing is obviously not okay. You'll also want to avoid very-polluted fish (like swordfish, tilefish, and shark), hydrogenated or partially hydrogenated oils (trans fats), and all artificial sweeteners. Soy and sugar are two other important ingredients to limit while nursing.

Soy. Soy contains plant-based estrogens that cause hormonal disruptions in both mom and nursing baby. Further, goitrogens (thyroid-blocking factors) in soy lead to metabolic problems and can make your thyroid underactive—leaving you exhausted, unable to lose weight, and with chilled fingers and toes. Additionally, children born to mothers with underactive thyroids have been found have IQs ten to fifteen points below average. (Learn more about soy's dangers in chapter 8.)

Sugars. Of all the problems with sugar, a major impact on your young baby is sugar's influence on yeast. When you eat sugars (table sugar, high fructose corn syrup, juice, white flour, etc.), you are feeding yeast (candida) in your body, allowing it to overgrow and potentially cause vaginal yeast infections, sugar cravings, and a painful breast infection called mastitis.

Though this ad is for Ovaltine, which has a sugar content and synthetic nutrients we don't recommend, it is interesting to recognize that even back in 1928, the quality of mom's diet was known to influence her milk quality and supply. As this ad says, "Statistics prove that a breast-fed baby's chances of living are increased 6 times . . . Here is a delightful way to a plentiful supply of natural milk . . ." With Super Nutrition, you don't need dietary supplemental beverages, just traditional foods, for a nutritious and adequate milk supply.

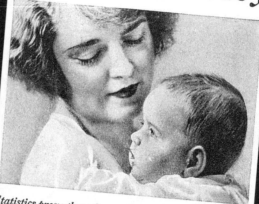

If you have yeast overgrowth in your gut, the yeast will likely pass to your baby and can result in thrush, diaper rash, food intolerances/food allergies, and nutrient deficiencies. When yeast eats sugar, it puts out toxic by-products that pass to your milk. In your baby's stomach, these by-products reduce her stomach acid. Since sufficient stomach acid is required to ward off acid reflux, related colic, food allergies, and even infection, it is wise to avoid eating sugar as a nursing mom.

Further, as your baby's immune system is developing, she is learning to differentiate between helpful and harmful flora. Your flora teaches her what is good and bad. If your baby is accustomed to getting yeast from you early in life, her body will likely perceive it as normal and allow it to thrive, thus potentially setting her up for a lifelong struggle with yeast-related issues such as sugar cravings, obesity, diabetes, mood/emotional disorders, asthma, allergies, alcoholism, and even heart disease.

MOM'S DRINKS

The most important advice for a nursing mom is to stay hydrated to provide enough fluid to produce milk. In fact, breast-feeding causes hormonal changes that can trigger incredible thirst during the first few minutes of a feeding—a built-in mechanism to ensure sufficient hydration. In addition to *how much* you drink, *what* you drink is also important both for you and your baby.

Caffeinated beverages. If you consume caffeine, be aware that it acts as a diuretic and can make you more prone to inadequate hydration, possibly affecting milk supply. Also, caffeine does get into breast milk, so watch for signs of caffeine sensitivity in your baby: wakefulness, hyperactivity, colicky behavior, and shorter duration of feedings. Caffeine comes from coffee, tea, chocolate, and soda pop.

In addition to being caffeinated, soda pop contains a metabolic nightmare of ingredients: high fructose corn syrup, as well as phosphates that block calcium and artificial flavorings and colorings. The artificial sweeteners in diet soda pop are unhealthy for anyone, particularly your baby.

Alcohol. You wouldn't feed your baby a martini in her bottle, so limit (or preferably cease) alcohol consumption while nursing. Alcohol enters breast milk 30 to 60 minutes after consumption. More than one or two social drinks can hinder "letdown" and can also create problems with sleep cycles in your baby. Feeling the effects of alcohol (an altered state) means alcohol is in your blood and equally in your milk. Wait at least 2 hours after any drink to nurse. If you have any more than one alcoholic drink, we advise you to "pump and dump."

Super Nutrition for Nursing Moms

As a nursing mom, you want your diet to contain as much nutrition as it can along with the least amount of toxins possible. (While this is sound advice for *everyone*, it is of particular importance when you've got the job of nourishing yourself *and* your baby!)

The Weston A. Price Foundation (WAPF) is a national non-profit nutrition organization and traditional-foods advocacy group. Founded in 1999, their experts have extensively studied the work of several researchers, who surmised from traditional, preindustrialized people that optimal health is entirely possible with the right form of foods and nutrient density. Based upon an extensive review of this research, WAPF has compiled and recommends a diet for pregnant and nursing mothers, as follows (reprinted with permission).

▸ Cod Liver Oil to supply* [no more than] 20,000 IU vitamin A and 2,000 IU vitamin D per day

▸ 1 quart (or 32 ounces [950 ml]) whole milk daily*, preferably raw and from pasture-fed cows (Learn more about raw milk on page 28.)

▸ 4 tablespoons (55 g) butter* daily, preferably from pasture-fed cows

▸ 2 or more eggs daily, preferably from pastured chickens

▸ Additional egg yolks daily, added to smoothies, salad dressings, scrambled eggs, etc.

▸ 3 to 4 ounces (85 to 115 g) fresh liver, once or twice per week

▸ Fresh seafood*, 2 to 4 times per week, particularly wild salmon, shellfish, and fish eggs

▸ Fresh beef or lamb daily, always consumed with the fat

▸ Oily fish* or lard daily, for vitamin D

▸ 2 tablespoons (28 g) coconut oil daily, used in cooking or smoothies, etc.

▸ Lacto-fermented condiments and beverages (see page 64)

▸ Bone broths used in soups, stews, and sauces

▸ Soaked [or sprouted] whole grains [and soaked or sprouted nuts and seeds] (page 136)

▸ Fresh vegetables and fruits

These recommendations are scientifically geared to nourish a nursing mother with all the minerals, enzymes, immune factors, vitamins, antioxidants, and fat-soluble activators she needs for herself and her baby. Many items should be consumed daily, but some should be a weekly goal. Below, we offer clarification on some of the guidelines, noted with (*) in the chart, as well as important information to best adapt them to your diet.

Vitamin A and cod liver oil. Taking cod liver oil (CLO) as a nursing mom provides benefits to both you and your baby. It is an excellent source of vitamins A and D, as well as the anti-inflammatory essential fatty acids DHA and EPA. The nutrients in CLO are in their most natural and "body-ready" form, making this single supplement extremely powerful in terms of health benefits. As for vitamin A, you'll get it predominantly from liver or cod liver oil, as well as *some* from eggs and butter. Though it is very, very important to get enough vitamin A, you don't want to exceed 20,000 IU per day. As a rule of thumb, if you eat liver, you don't necessarily need to take cod liver oil that day.

All that milk! Thirty-two ounces (950 ml) of milk is equal to *four big glasses*. If the milk you're drinking is fresh, raw, and grass fed, your hardworking, nursing body will likely love it. If you don't have access to a clean, raw dairy, hold off on drinking that much, as pasteurized milk is often irritating and inflammatory. To minimize inflammation and maximize nutrition, choose milk that is organic, preferably grass fed, nonhomogenized, and vat pasteurized (lower heat); see WAPF shopping guide in Resources (page 218), for brands. Or instead, combine some high-quality whole-milk plain yogurt (8 to 16 ounces, or 225 to 455 g) and cheese (about 4 ounces, or 115 g) daily, and make sure you get Souper Stock (page 56) several times per week, if not daily, as well.

Cod Liver Oil Is Not the Same as Fish Oil

Fish *liver* oils are whole-food-based supplements that are rich in important nutrients. If fermented, these oils are also a source of vitamin K2. Further, high-quality cod *liver* oil provides the right ratios of fat-soluble, mineral-activating vitamins and essential fatty acids ratios. Fish oil contains *only* omega-3 fatty acids, without the important vitamins A and D.

If you suspect your baby is irritated by the pasteurized dairy you are consuming, we urge you to procure a source of trusted raw dairy. (Refer to "Got Raw?" on page 28.) But if raw dairy is truly inaccessible, we suggest Souper Stock *with each meal*, daily, to attempt to provide the absorbable minerals that would've been found in dairy in your diet. Additionally, probiotics and cod liver oil are a must in the absence of high-quality dairy. Usually, butter is tolerable (and desirable!), even if pasteurized milk is not; but if not, we recommend ghee.

Does it have to be whole milk? Yes, whole milk is a whole food. Stripping away the fat does far more than just reduce the calories. Important nutrients, including vitamins A and D, in milk are housed in the fat. These vitamins need to be consumed with fat to be used by the body, and without them, you can't use the minerals in the foods you eat either. Whole (or unchanged) milk provides fat, fat-soluble vitamins, and minerals—all of which work together. (Remember, nursing burns calories, and fat is satisfying, so don't worry that you'll "overindulge"!)

Butter—Better than you thought! Butter from grass-fed cows is an amazing healing food. Grass-fed, raw butter contains fat-soluble vitamin A (retinol), fat-soluble beta-carotene, conjugated linoleic acid (a potent cancer-fighting fat found almost exclusively in grass-fed dairy and animal fat), omega-3s (which are crucial to building your baby's brain, like DHA), and fat-soluble vitamin E. Several fatty acids in butter support the immune, digestive, and nervous system. High-quality butter is a Super POWER food because it provides such excellent nutrients, along with the fat to make sure your body can use them! No longer should you view butter as a stick of fat, but as a great source of nourishment, which just so happens to also make foods taste great! Additionally, though we unnecessarily fear saturated fat, the nutrients in grass-fed, organic butter (particularly raw), have so many benefits, it is undeniably a heart- and health-*helpful* food.

Seafood safety. We recommend *wild-caught* seafood, but in instances where you can be assured no antibiotics, vaccines, or GMO feed are used, then high-quality farm-raised is acceptable. To reduce heavy metal and pollutant risk, we strongly recommend that at least half of the two to four weekly fish servings come from small, oily fish (such as sardines or anchovies) or fish roe (caviar), which are the least contaminated.

ANIMAL AND SEA FOODS

We urge you to consume plenty of animal foods, as well as some sea foods. The source of the animal foods you eat, though, and what *they* ate, is very important. Pastured, grass-fed animal foods are the very best. Next best is organic. Less nutritious is "all natural." Finally, you've got conventional, or "normal", animal foods at your regular grocery store.

THE RIGHT FATS

Your milk is made of high quantities of saturated fat and cholesterol, which are essential to your baby's development, most importantly her brain development. Your milk is naturally made of close to 60 percent fat and cholesterol, almost identical to the fat content of babies' brains—also made of about 60 percent fat. If you don't provide your body with enough fat and cholesterol in your diet, your body will be taxed with making them for your milk. (If you never eat saturated fat, your body will make this important nutrient from carbohydrates. But why tax enzymes and nutrients to do this? Just supply some in your diet.)

Fabulous Fats

All fats—saturated and unsaturated—are 9 calories per gram. Vegetable fats are not "lower fat" than fats in steak, and fats in bacon are no "fattier" than fats from corn, soybeans, or cottonseed. If anything, vegetable oils may be more likely to contribute to fat storage. According to Alan Greene, M.D., in *Feeding Baby Green*, vegetable fats are inflammatory and consequently slow down the body's fat-burning capabilities, contributing to fat storage and thus, weight gain. Following are some of the myriad benefits of animal fats.

Butter helps with cholesterol metabolism, growth, and glucose tolerance; promotes healthy bones and teeth; aids metabolic and biochemical pathways; builds the brain; and fights free radicals, toxins, cancer, infection, and inflammation. If it is raw and grass fed, it helps prevent arthritis and calcification of the arteries. Farm-fresh is best, organic is great, but even "regular" butter is better than any "spreads."

Ghee is clarified butter and is typically safe for those who react to the milk protein casein. Ghee still has all the vitamins of butter, but some factors found in raw butter are lost.

Lard is mostly a monounsaturated fat, like olive oil. If it comes from pastured pigs, then their fat is an excellent source of vitamin D (containing twelve times more than conventional pork fat). To render lard, see the recipe on page 187.

Rendered chicken fat (schmaltz). Chicken fat can also be rendered and used for sautéing (see Schmaltz and Gribenes recipe on page 113). Chicken fat contains palmitoleic fatty acid—an antimicrobial (immune-supporting) fat.

Beef suet and tallow. Suet (fat from the cavity of the animal) is predominantly saturated fat, so it's a great fat for high heat. Tallow, the rendered fat, is just over half saturated fat and about 40 percent monounsaturated. Both can be used for frying and have antimicrobial (immune-boosting) fatty acids. Often suet and tallow can be found at local farms.

Marrow. Archaeological digs reveal bones that were cracked and broken to extract the precious and nutritious marrow inside. Bone marrow is an "organ" that is mostly made of fat. It contains nutrients not found in muscle meat and has iron, vitamin A, phosphorus, and unique AKGs (alkylglycerols)—which are special fats that boost the immune system.

Coconut oil and red palm oil. Second only to mom's milk, coconut oil is an excellent source of virus-fighting lauric acid. It is also remarkably rich in special fatty acids that help with keeping the gut healthy and that don't like to turn into body fat. Coconut oil is great support for the thyroid gland—the master of metabolism.

Red palm oil is a stable fat great for high-heat cooking. Extremely rich in antioxidants, it provides all eight kinds of vitamin E and four kinds of carotenes, as well as more lycopene and lutein than tomatoes and carrots combined—all of which require fat to be absorbed and used, making this fat a superior source of them. It is great for frying (particularly for making sprouted tortillas into homemade chips!).

Proper proportion of fats. Most of your fats should come from butter, eggs, cheese, and meat. Coconut fats (oil and milk) should contribute significantly to your fat intake, due to their special medium-chain triglycerides (fats that help feed probiotics, spur metabolism, and lend themselves to healthy thyroid function). Fish, oily fish, and nuts will round out essential fatty acid needs.

Heating and proper usage. Heat, light, time, pressure, and chemicals damage fats, but some are more vulnerable to rancidity than others. Rancid fats are dangerous, contribute to oxidative stress, use nutrient and antioxidant stores, and are a significant source of disease-causing free radicals. Polyunsaturated fats are most vulnerable, whereas saturated fats are the least susceptible. All oils should be cold-pressed and unrefined, if possible. Below describes various kinds of fats and their best cooking applications (despite what their label might say) and heat tolerances.

▸ **Saturated fats:** coconut oil, butter, ghee, red palm oil, or palm kernel oil; use for sautéing at high heat. Such fats are solid at room temperature and are molecularly stable enough to withstand damage from high heat. Best baking fats include butter, ghee (butter oil), and lard.

▸ **Combination saturated/monounsaturated fats:** Fats that are saturated, monounsaturated, and polyunsaturated, such as suet and beef tallow, lard, or schmaltz are best used at medium-high heat.

▸ **Predominantly monounsaturated fats:** olive oil, avocado oil, hazelnut oil, macadamia nut oil, high-oleic safflower oil, and almond oil; can handle moderate heat, so use in medium- to low-heat cooking.

▸ **Combination monounsaturated and polyunsaturated fats:** peanut oil and pumpkin seed oil; these can be used in medium-low-heat cooking, like light sautéing. Sesame oil is both mono- and polyunsaturated fat but has antioxidant factors (sesamin) that make it better able to handle moderate heat than other combination mono- and polyunsaturates.

▸ **Polyunsaturated fats:** walnut oil, flaxseed oil, perilla seed oil, and borage oil; these are great for cold applications of oils, like salad dressings, and need protection (from heat, light, and time). They should be kept in dark bottles, stored in the refrigerator. Polyunsaturates should make up the lowest portion of your fat intake

WISE CARBS

As for carbohydrates, eat a variety of greens, vegetables, fruits, nuts, and seeds. We call these "wise" carbs because they pack much more nutrition and fiber—and don't spike your blood sugar as much—as the more commonly consumed carbs, such as refined grains, beans, and tubers. Grains and beans need special preparation to make them most nutritious because without such preparation, they block nutrients and are hard on the digestive tract. (Refer to chapter 6 for a discussion on preparing grains and legumes properly.)

Supplements for Mom and Babe

Before you brought your baby home from the hospital or birthing center, you were likely advised to continue taking your prenatal vitamins if you're breast-feeding. We do think it's a good idea to take supplements while nursing, in general, but must point out that it is never enough to provide you with what you need to maintain your own health, let alone that of your baby, so your diet remains of utmost importance. Below are the supplements we recommend for you, as well as the special circumstances where your baby might also need supplements.

RECOMMENDED SUPPLEMENTS FOR YOU

The dietary recommendations we've given, as well as the guidelines from the Weston A. Price Foundation, are an ideal *goal*. As we realize that you may not consume all these foods on a regular basis, we recommend supplements to fill in the blanks (see Resources for ordering information). We recommend nursing moms take the following *daily*:

Multivitamin. If your diet is close to our dietary recommendations for nursing moms, you won't need a multi. However, if you are working toward such a diet, and still aren't there yet, you might be wise to take a multivitamin or prenatal vitamin. We strongly advise taking a 100 percent food-based vitamin and mineral supplement (you can ask for this at your health food store) or at least a high-quality synthetic supplement (again, rely on your local health food store or trusted healthcare provider).

Cod liver oil. If not fermented cod liver oil, then take high-quality cod liver oil *plus* high-vitamin butter oil, following the dosage recommendations on the bottle.

Liver. If you don't eat liver, we recommend taking desiccated liver: Six pills should be equivalent to 1 ounce (28 g) of liver.

Probiotics. We recommend probiotics for many reasons (see "Power Up Immunity with Plentiful Probiotics," page 96). Typically, a capsule or two per night is appropriate. Ten to 20 billion colonizing forming units (CFUs) is adequate (though too many isn't a concern). A multistrain formula of probiotics is best, as each person's bacterial makeup is as individual as her fingerprint. Ensure that your probiotic contains *Lactobacillus acidophilus* and *Bifidobacterium*.

Vitamin D3. Nursing mothers and their babies benefit from vitamin D3 doses higher than the 1,000 IU per day recommended by most OB/GYNs, except moms who get plenty of midday sunlight or frequently eat fish roe. Studies show moms taking 6,400 IU vitamin D3 per day provide breast milk levels of 873 IU/L. Thus, a daily dose of 5,000 to 6,000 IU of vitamin D3 with 1 teaspoon of cod liver oil (containing 400 IU of vitamin D) is ideal, and no vitamin supplementation is necessary for your baby. There can be significant variability between people with regard to ideal vitamin D dosing. Since vitamin D is a fat-soluble vitamin, it can accumulate, so it is best to get your blood level for vitamin D checked (ask your doctor for the 25-OHD3 test) every 3 months after starting high-dose vitamin D with a target level between 60 to 80; once you get to that level,

Vitamin D Is Essential for Health

Vitamin D is critical for everyone, from fetuses to the elderly. Inadequate vitamin D levels are found to increase the risk of nearly every illness that exists, from both types of diabetes, asthma, and multiple sclerosis, to heart disease and cancer. By supplementing vitamin D, the risk of overall illness decreases, and even small increases in vitamin D levels have been shown to make a positive impact. Research shows that when moms have enough vitamin D, babies have better birth weights, larger head circumferences, better tooth enamel, and less asthma and allergies. If newborns have good vitamin D levels, they'll have increased bone mass at birth and better bone mineralization for at least 9 years, which safeguards against rickets, osteopenia (low bone mineral density), and fractures.

you can reduce your vitamin D intake by half and verify that it is remaining high at your next blood check. Note: More vitamin D is usually needed in winter months, when less sun exposure is available.

Folic acid. This vitamin is vital to the function of our biochemical pathways and detoxification. Practitioners like Dr. Amy Yasko, who has her Ph.D. in microbiology, immunology, and infectious disease and works closely with autistic and other chronically ill children, are finding that the majority of people with illness have difficulty with efficiently processing folic acid, derived either from food or from supplementation. In our world so full of toxins, detoxification is critical in maintaining good health. Thus, to maximize health, we recommend moms take 1 mg daily of a special form of folic acid, called 5-methyltetrahydrafolate ("5-MTHF" for short). As B12 assists this pathway, we encourage getting plenty of B12 from animal foods (liver, meat, fish, eggs, and dairy).

RECOMMENDED SUPPLEMENTS FOR YOUR BABY

With your stellar diet and additional supplements, it is unlikely that your baby needs supplementation during these first 6 months. There are, however, some circumstances that call for them.

Probiotics. Give supplemental probiotics to your baby if:
- Your baby was born by C-section.
- You had antibiotics during pregnancy, delivery, or while nursing.
- You or your baby were given steroids or antibiotics.
- You have a history of yeast infections or had a yeast infection during pregnancy.

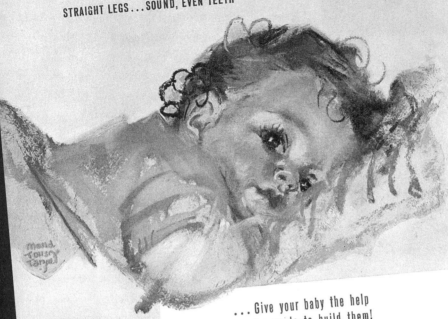

A WELL-SHAPED HEAD...A FINE, FULL CHEST...A STRONG BACK

STRAIGHT LEGS...SOUND, EVEN TEETH

... Give your baby the help he needs to build them!

His important first year! Your baby's head grows as much as it will the rest of his life. He'll sit up alone. Then later, he will walk! How necessary to provide plenty of Vitamin D to help him build the *right kind* of head, back, chest, legs. Millions of mothers rely on Squibb Cod Liver Oil as a dependable source of Vitamin D. See that *your* baby gets it daily!

Triple his birth weight!.....Your baby may weigh three times as much at the end of 12 months as at birth. But there are other signs to check. Is he sitting up erect? (Grown-up posture may depend on the framework he builds now.) Is his chest well-developed? Are his legs growing straight? To help him build a good framework, give him Squibb Cod Liver Oil as part of a well-balanced diet.

Teeth coming through?.....Remember Vitamin D helps baby transform the calcium and phosphorus he gets from food into sound tooth structure. When those first teeth come in the right way—sound and not too close together—there is plenty of room later for permanent teeth to develop properly. Another reason for giving Squibb Cod Liver Oil, an excellent source of Vitamin D.

Daily use important!.....The sun gives baby less than one-fourth the Vitamin D protection in mid-winter as in early summer. He can't get much Vitamin D from sunshine indoors. Cloudy weather, clothing shut out much of the sunlight. Food may not make up this vitamin loss. So many physicians advise starting Squibb Cod Liver Oil soon after birth.

Vitamins guarded! You get what you pay for!
When you insist on Squibb Cod Liver Oil for your baby, you get *full value* of the vitamins A and D you are paying for. Squibb Cod Liver Oil provides more than twice as many units of Vitamin A and three times as much Vitamin D as a cod liver oil which meets minimum requirements of the U.S. Pharmacopeia. *Specially tested* for vitamins. Exceptionally potent.....You'll find the Squibb oil an economy! At any drug store.

SQUIBB *Cod Liver Oil*   *The priceless ingredient of every product is the honor and integrity of its maker*

◄ In 1940, this advertisement made bold boasts about the benefits of providing cod liver oil to children: "a well-shaped head . . . a fine, full chest . . . a strong back, straight legs . . . sound, even teeth. Give your baby the help he needs to build them." These claims are actually very true; we now know more about the fat-soluble mineral activators found in cod liver oil: vitamins A and D3. These nutrients—sadly lacking in our modern children's diet—ensure minerals are usable such that skeletal structure is optimized. Additionally, brain growth and cognitive development rely on special Omega-3 fatty acids such as DHA found in cod liver oil. Such wisdom from generations ago—lost over the last several decades—should again come to the forefront. Particularly during the first year of rapid growth, the unique, natural nutrients in cod liver oil are a splendid way to help your child's busily growing body and brain to develop.

A Word about Sweeteners

It is very important to limit sweets, but those you do include should come from whole foods because they are able to offer some nutrient value.

- Dehydrated whole sugar cane (Rapunzel brand "Rapadura")
- Blackstrap molasses
- Honey (raw, unheated, unfiltered)
- Maple syrup (pure, grade B or lower)
- Date sugar
- Coconut palm sugar—100 percent pure only
- Carob (rather than chocolate)
- Stevia—whole plant (Sweetleaf brand green powder or brown liquid)
- Erythritol sweetened with luo han guo fruit is called Lankanto and is a nonglycemic sweetener that can be used in baking (available only at www.bodyecology.com)

▸ Your baby has thrush or a yeast diaper rash.
▸ You or your family has a history of alcoholism, sugar cravings, diabetes, metabolic syndrome, or other sugar-related illnesses.

(For more information about this important supplement, see Power Up Immunity with Plentiful Probiotics, page 96). Powdered-probiotics baby dosing is about 3 billion CFU/day, but more importantly, pay attention to the strains specifically *Lactobacillus acidophilus* and *Bifidobacterium infantis* (aka *Bifidobacterium animalis*), and choose the highest quality brand you can. Probiotics can be given by simply putting ¼ teaspoon on your wet finger and letting your baby suck it off or by putting it on your nipple during nursing once or twice a day. Probiotics can also be added to the contents of a bottle, though you risk losing some, as they can get stuck coating the interior of the bottle.

Cod liver oil. In most cases, the cod liver oil you are taking will provide the most nutritious milk for your baby. In certain circumstances, including sibling or parental history of a 3C condition, it might be wise to provide CLO directly. For dosing and administration information for your baby, see page 59.

Vitamin D. A nursing baby will only need additional vitamin D if you are taking less than 5,000 IU per day, in which case he should be supplemented with 400 IU per day. (See Resources for brands.)

Recipes for Nursing Moms and Their Families

The ultimate resource for the most nutritious and most digestible foods is *Nourishing Traditions* by Sally Fallon, author, researcher, traditional-foods advocate, and founder and president of the Weston A. Price Foundation. We've adapted several of her recipes throughout this book, with permission. Though these recipes are ideal for nursing mamas, we feel they're extremely beneficial to the health of your entire family—including your baby, where noted. (You can also enjoy the recipes recommended for your baby throughout the book; they are nutritious for you as well as for her!)

Regarding the animal foods mentioned in the recipes, it is implied that animal foods are the highest quality available to you, either from a farm co-op (refer to page 52 for more information), an Internet order, a health food store, or are at least organic and free of most chemicals and minimally processed.

Fish Roe Spreads

Fish roe is extremely nutritious and held sacred for its health properties around the world. Mix fish roe into mayonnaise, pesto, egg salad, or with sour cream and green onions. Or use fish roe as a garnish. Feed these spreads to your baby after 1 year of age, too!

Pineapple Chutney

Pineapples are a sweet treat—and as a tropical fruit are great at digesting themselves! By allowing good bacteria to feed on their sugars, their available nutrition is escalated. This tasty dish, adapted from Nourishing Traditions *by Sally Fallon, is suitable for your baby after age one.*

2 cups (310 g) diced pineapple (from whole, fresh pineapple)

¼ cup (60 ml) filtered water

Juice of ½ lemon or lime

2 tablespoons (28 ml) whey (see Homemade Whey, page 64)

¼ teaspoon Celtic sea salt

½ bunch finely chopped cilantro

Mix all the ingredients in a mason jar. Tamp down the pineapple under the water (add more water if needed). Leave for 24 hours, sealed on the counter.

Yield: Approximately ½ quart (475 ml)

Notes

- This is a great side dish to serve with wild-caught fish; cilantro is known to block toxic mercury from being absorbed.
- It may be stored in the refrigerator for 2 months.

Fried Veggie Fritters

This is a yummy way to eat your veggies. It's perfect to serve your baby after age 1.

1 cup (245 g) cooked puréed vegetables (zucchini, sweet potatoes, pumpkin, or parsnips)

½ finely chopped small onion

1 egg

¼ cup (32 g) arrowroot starch

Celtic sea salt, to taste

2 to 3 tablespoons (28 to 45 g) butter, ghee, (26 to 39 g) lard, or (28 to 45 ml)olive oil

Mix the ingredients, minus the fat, in a bowl. Form into palm-size patties.

Warm the fat in a frying pan over medium-high heat. Saute the fritters and flip until golden.

Yield: 4 to 6 fritters

Note

- Serve topped with Apple Spread (page 161) or roe spread (page 183).

Banana Cream Custard

This delicious and nutritious special-occasion treat is adapted from Nourishing a Growing Baby *by Jen Allbritton. Make it for your baby after 1 year of age.*

1 cup (235 ml) milk (whole cow's, whole goat's, raw, coconut, even mom's if you're game)

½ cup (120 ml) cream—raw preferred

1 small, brown-spotted banana,

6 egg yolks

½ teaspoon vanilla extract

Pinch of stevia, optional

Preheat the oven to 310°F (154°C).

Mix all the ingredients together. Pour the mixture into four 6-ounce (175 ml) buttered ramekins.

Place the ramekins into an 8 × 8-inch (20 × 20 cm) glass baking dish and fill the dish with water until it comes halfway up the sides of the ramekins.

Cook for 1 hour until the custards are set.

Yield: 4 custards

Enzyme-Boost Smoothie

Foods containing enzymes reduce the body's burden of making its own. Often, when you add more enzyme-rich foods to your diet, your metabolic function improves and your energy will perk up. Your baby might enjoy this with you after age 7 months.

1 fresh chopped mango + ½ cup (115 g) ice (or 2 cups [350 g] packaged frozen mango)

1 large or 2 small brown-spotted bananas

¼ cup (60 ml) unsweetened coconut water, plus more to thin

½ avocado

Purée in a blender until desired consistency.

Yield: About 2 cups (475 ml)

Note

- Mixture can be frozen for a summer treat.

Coconut Tonic

This tonic, from Eat Fat Lose Fat *by Mary Enig, Ph.D., and Sally Fallon, is nutritious and mineral rich, as well as tasty and tummy-friendly. You can serve this to your baby in limited quantities after 1 year of age.*

1 can (8 ounces, or 235 ml) coconut milk

2¼ cups (535 ml) water

2 tablespoons (40 g) maple syrup or pinch whole plant stevia

1 teaspoon vanilla extract

1 teaspoon dolomite powder

Mix the ingredients in a medium saucepan and cook over medium-low heat.
Heat until warm and the dolomite is dissolved. Serve warm.

Yield: About 1 quart (950 ml)

Notes

- Be sure purchase only KAL brand dolomite powder with a USP label to minimize the chances of lead contamination.
- Drink this for a nutritious treat, as a "pick-me-up," or to soothe your digestive tract before or during illness.

Mom to Mom / Studies show that babies will stay at the breast longer if their moms have had vanilla or garlic. Avoid alcohol, bitter flavors, and coffee—since these have been shown to shorten the time a baby will stay at the breast.

Kombucha

Kombucha is made by fermenting tea by use of a SCOBY (symbiotic culture of bacteria and yeast). The scoby is "fed" sugar and floats in the tea. The microbes eat the sugars, and the resulting fermented tea is a source of amino acids, organic acids, enzymes, and probiotics. An ounce or two (28 to 60 ml) of this digestive aid with each meal is wonderful. You can serve this to your baby in small quantities (1 to 2 ounces [28 to 60 ml]) with meals after 1 year of age, as some small amount of natural alcohol may be produced through fermentation. Order a kombucha kit from www.happyherbalist.com to make your own or purchase kombucha from your health food store. Just watch the sugar content. There should be 2 to 3 grams of sugar per serving. Anything more, and the scoby is fed more sugar than it can eat, which results in a sugary beverage for you (or your baby)—not ideal.

Shoot for high-quality, grass-fed, organic, aged beef. You'll reap the following benefits:

- The stearic acid in steak is converted in the body to oleic acid, the healthy, coveted fatty acid in olive oil.
- Red meat, from grass-fed animals, is a good source of omega-3s and vitamin E.
- Red meat is a rich source of nutrients, including B6, zinc, phosphorus, carnitine, CoQ10, and B1, that protect the heart and nervous system.

Several studies have shown that higher-fat, lower-carb diets result in more weight loss, better heart health markers, improved insulin sensitivity, and lower blood glucose than do high-carb, low-fat diets.

Interestingly, the taurine, carnitine, and CoQ10 found in red meat are superbly powerful in ensuring and restoring healthy cardiovascular function. A grass-fed steak might be just what the doctor *should* order for heart health!

Nut 'n' Honey Balls

Honey—if unfiltered, unheated, and raw—is a nutritious, natural sweetener. It contains amylase, so it aids carbohydrate digestion. The honey will work on digesting starches if you allow it to work on the foods it is mixed with for 15 minutes or so before eating it (as with oatmeal). A good snack for you, this can be a terrific special occasion treat for your baby over 1 year.

1 cup (260 g) soaked nut butter (page 137)

1 cup (104 g) sprouted seeds (page 136), ground in a coffee grinder or food processer

½ cup (170 g) raw, unheated, unfiltered honey

½ cup (43 g) unsweetened, unsulfured, shredded coconut

Stir together the nut butter, seeds, and honey. Mix well.

Roll the mixture into 1-inch (2.5 cm) balls. Roll the balls in the coconut.

Yield: 10 to 12 balls

Zucchini Fries

A more nutritious option than white-potato-based fries (particularly those from frozen or fast-food places), these zucchini fries are great for tired moms who want a treat!

2 medium zucchini

2 tablespoons (28 ml) milk (human, cow, or coconut)

1 egg, lightly beaten

¼ cup (32 g) arrowroot starch

½ cup (about 50 g) fresh grated cheese (preferably raw)

¼ cup (21 g) unsweetened, unsulfured shredded coconut

Garlic powder to taste

Celtic sea salt to taste

3 tablespoons (42 g) butter or (39 g) lard

Cut the zucchini in half and then into small, fry-length spears. Mix the milk and egg until combined. Combine the arrowroot, cheese, coconut, garlic powder, and salt in a small bowl or pie plate. Dip the spears in the milk-egg mixture and roll the spears the arrowroot mixture. Warm the butter or lard in a frying pan over medium heat. Add the coated zucchini fries and cook until golden, turning with tongs.

Yield: About 36 "fries"

Note

- You can also bake the "fries" for 25 minutes at 400°F (200°C, gas mark 6) on a greased cookie sheet.

Lard

Put unrendered leaf lard (the fat from around the kidneys), as procured from a local farm, in a pot, pan, or slow cooker (no water) on low. Once every half hour, flip it with tongs and pierce the white sections, which should liquefy in the warmth. Not everything will turn to liquid; you'll be left with brown "cracklin" (which is tasty with sea salt). When no or few white parts remain, it is done. Strain into a glass container to cool on your counter. The rendered lard will turn white as it cools. You can leave some out and store the rest in the refrigerator. Used with sea salt, it's great for potatoes.

Nursing and Feeding Advice

Many experts call the first 3 months after birth the "fourth trimester," which implies that babies require time to transition into the outside world. Your baby isn't familiar with stillness, quiet, or fabric surroundings. Comfort is found in you—your voice, breathing, gait, smell, and the rhythm of your heartbeat. Talk softly to her, try skin to skin contact or swaddle her tightly (especially if she is fussy), and gently rock her or carry her as you walk. Your baby is used to a nearly constant source of nutrition; to mimic that as much as possible, allow her to eat any time she is hungry (breast-fed babies *need* to eat frequently).

Get in sync with your baby. Your baby's sucking frequency significantly dictates your milk production. Your body's goal is to make exactly how much milk your baby needs, and it is your baby's act of sucking that provides this information. Nurse too infrequently and your body thinks your baby doesn't need very much; nurse too frequently (like pumping in between feedings) and your body thinks you have twins and overproduces. By letting your baby be the *sole guide* for your body for the first 2 weeks, you'll get in perfect synchronization with her, providing her with plenty of nourishment without overproducing and engorgement.

Feed on cue. Rather than clock-watching, we recommend you tune in to your baby. When she signals, with simple alertness, rooting, mouthing, physical activity, or any other sign that you interpret as a message to you, let her nurse. The AAP states, "During the early weeks of breast-feeding, mothers should be encouraged to . . . [offer] the breast *whenever* the infant shows *early* signs of hunger." Crying, the AAP says, "is a *late* indicator of hunger." [emphases added]

Rather than calling this "on demand," we prefer to call it "on cue." "Demand" implies that your baby is bossing you around, which couldn't be further from the truth. "Cues," on the other hand, signify the very special nonverbal communication that occurs between mother and child. (Note: Cues are easily missed when you aren't holding your baby, as when she's in a carrier, crib, swing, bouncy, or you're otherwise apart.)

When formula is not necessarily necessary. In the first few days, parents often have concerns that their baby not getting enough milk. Be reassured that frequent nursing and weight loss are both to be expected. Your newborn's hunger drives her to nurse frequently, which stimulates your milk to come in. In most cases, encouraging formula feeding is counterproductive to nursing and can further decrease milk supply. Though your milk hasn't yet come in, colostrum, the early yellowish, thick liquid that is present before "mature" milk comes in, is the ultimate protective nutrition—your baby needs nothing more. Colostrum is very rich in nutrients, probiotics, and immune factors. The human baby is *designed* to feed *first* on colostrum for several days before having *anything* else; the colostrum actually prepares your baby's gut to digest the coming milk.

SPECIAL FEEDING CONCERNS

Stress and anxiety can interfere with digestion because they shift nutrients and blood away from digestive functions. Studies show that when your baby is being held by you, pain-relieving endorphins (the body's internal morphine) are released by her brain. If your baby is experiencing tummy trouble, fear, chill, loneliness, anxiety, or other distress, holding her literally dulls or takes away her pain and discomfort. Minimizing your baby's stress by holding her continuously and making eye contact, particularly as you nurse her, is important for emotional and digestive health.

Tummy trouble (gas). Commonly, foods that cause gas in you can cause gas in your baby, namely raw, fibrous greens and veggies; some fruits; and onions, grains, and beans. If your baby is gassy, cook all fruits and vegetables you eat and prepare grains and beans as described in chapter 6. It is also helpful to consume enzyme- and probiotic-rich foods such as any of the lacto-fermented foods or beverages found in this chapter or others.

More Serious Concerns

If your baby isn't growing in length or head circumference, is losing weight, *or* she isn't nursing enough, you *should* have real concerns. Failure to thrive or not growing at all can represent more serious problems. *If your instincts tell you something is wrong, follow them, regardless of what your pediatrician says.* Lack of gain in head circumference can be related to B12 deficiency if mom is not getting adequate animal foods. Please see our dietary recommendations for nursing moms to ensure adequate B12 (and other critical nutrients) for your baby, page 171.

Colic from acid reflux. Colic, or excessive and unreasonable crying, occurs in one out of every four infants. Though the cause of colic is unknown, colic is often thought to be due to reflux or some other cause of pain. If painful acid reflux is the cause of your baby's discomfort and colic, we advise you to eat adequate probiotic-rich foods and take a probiotic supplement. Avoiding sugar and refined grains helps to minimize unhealthy microbes in your gut (and their toxic by-products) that can lead to digestive distress in your baby. Include lactic acid–rich foods in your diet, like unpasteurized pickles or sauerkraut (or other lacto-fermented foods or cultured dairy—see page 64). It may also be beneficial to directly supplement your baby with probiotics (see page 180). If painful reflux persists despite taking these measures, unpasteurized sauerkraut juice (¼ teaspoon or less) given directly to your baby at the beginning of a meal might be helpful.

Colic from too much sugar, not enough fat. The duration of a feeding will influence the quality of nutrition your baby receives. If she is getting too much lactose (in foremilk, the milk in the early part of a feeding) without adequate fat (from hindmilk, which comes later), the milk sugar will ferment in her gut, creating gas. This leads to fussiness and colic symptoms. Your baby needs the fat that comes at the end of the feeding. Allow your baby to nurse for as long as she desires on one breast and *only then* switch to the other. This should ensure the right balance of foremilk to hindmilk, helping to resolve discomfort that may result from a "low-fat" diet.

Drugstore Formula Doesn't Cut It

Better Options Than Commercial Alternatives

For those who cannot or choose not to breast-feed, commercial formula is commonly accepted as the safest— and only—alternative for infants. Even breast-fed babies may, for a variety of reasons, be fed infant formulas at some point during their first year. How your baby is nourished is especially important when he isn't exclusively nursed, so we've dedicated particular attention to providing you with better options than just the commercial, powdered corn syrup and vegetable oil–based formulas on the grocery and drugstore shelves. This chapter will provide you with several alternatives so that you can better balance your baby's nutritional needs with your time, resources, and budgetary constraints.

The Very Real Risks of Commercial Formula

Ever wonder why they call it "formula"? During the last century and a half, some serious mistakes have been made in formula recipes, leaving out critical nutrients and constituents that babies need for survival and proper growth and development. The "formula" for formula still isn't perfected, and several risks are involved in commercial formula feeding.

> **Mom to Mom /** Starting as early as 4 months, depending on your baby's ready-to-eat signs, babies fed commercial formula benefit from earlier feeding of nutritious first foods (see chapter 2).

UNHEALTHY INGREDIENTS

Reading the label on most formula containers might set off health-conscious warning bells, as many of the ingredients are clearly not nutritious choices: corn syrup, inflammatory oils, genetically modified foods, and synthetic nutrients. Unfortunately, most people don't read the ingredients on the canister of formula. If you have a canister in your cupboard, go ahead and take a look now.

UNACCEPTABLE SAFETY STANDARDS

In the United States, formula ingredients must only meet Generally Recognized as Safe (GRAS) status. This is a category that was developed to regulate food ingredients for the *general population*, "*not* for infants who are a more vulnerable population," [emphasis added] as is stated in a report prepared for the FDA and Health Canada in 2004, "Infant Formula: Evaluating the Safety of New Ingredients." With regard to getting GRAS status, there is a significant conflict of interest because it is up to the manufacturer to declare the ingredient safe; no independent agency evaluation is required.

LACKING IN LIVING ORGANISMS

Commercial formula lacks probiotics, prebiotics, and the living immune cells found in mom's milk that support the gut and the immune system. Though some formula manufacturers have begun to add probiotics to formula, they require specific living conditions to survive, and they are only beneficial when alive. Unfortunately, testing done on many products claiming to contain probiotics frequently proves them to be dead and therefore of no benefit whatsoever.

WRONG SUGARS CAN HINDER DIGESTION AND BRAIN DEVELOPMENT

Lactose is the main carbohydrate source in human milk, cow's milk, and cow's milk–based formula. As the easiest sugar for your baby to digest, lactose breaks down into glucose and galactose; the latter is instrumental in brain building. Lactose is therefore the only sugar your infant should ingest. Soy and lactose-free formulas, however, use other sugars (like corn syrup) that cause sugar and insulin spikes, followed by crashes that are disruptive to the body; this differs from lactose, which releases energy steadily. Alternative sweeteners don't offer any galactose and instead break down into glucose and *fructose.* Joseph Mercola, M.D., best-selling author and featured medical expert on several major news channels, reports that "many infant formulas have as much or more high fructose corn syrup than a can of soda."

COMPETING NUTRIENTS

Formula's nutrients can block each other, making the formula not as nutritious in reality as it reads on the label. Also, adding new ingredients to formulas can change the requirements for competing nutrients. For example, iron was added to soy formula because soy's natural phytic acid blocked iron from being absorbed. Then, because iron absorption was still poor, vitamin C was added as an attempt to improve absorption. Iron and vitamin C together then blocked both copper and zinc. Recently, formula companies are adding more zinc to try to compensate.

Though minimum nutrient standards are set, unfortunately, no testing is required to ensure that all necessary nutrient levels are reached considering combinations. Most often, formula manufacturers overlook such nutrient relationships. Surprisingly, the FDA does not approve infant formulas before they're sold to the public. The FDA must simply be notified before the new formula is introduced. This is quite concerning, as some ingredients, when combined, can lead to toxicity in addition to imbalances in important nutrients.

Seemingly beneficial nutrient additions can cause such ripple effects in terms of changing requirements for other nutrients that the process must be cautiously reviewed. Improving formula requires a thorough understanding of the nuances of Nature's interactions between nutrients, and even our best scientists simply do not have a full grasp of such complexities. Trying to recreate Nature is a bit like chasing your tail.

CONTAMINANTS AND RECALLS

Mass manufacturing of commercial formula too often results in residues, pollutants, infestations, and other contaminant problems that have led to recalls. In the fall of 2010, many Similac varieties were voluntarily recalled after "identifying a common warehouse beetle (both larvae and adults) in the finished product," according to the FDA.

TOXINS

In 2008, one of China's infant formulas was found to have melamine contamination, sickening more than 50,000 babies and resulting in four deaths; traces were found in U.S. formula, as well, putting babies in danger of significant kidney disease. While claimed to be accidental, it is speculated that melamine was added to falsely elevate protein levels. In 2009, the CDC discovered perchlorate—a toxic compound used in rocket fuel—in fifteen brands of infant formula, including the two best-selling brands.

Even the packaging isn't safe. The inside lining of formula containers often contains bisphenol A (BPA). BPA is a toxin that acts as an endocrine disruptor and is linked to learning disabilities and reproductive changes. The European Safety Authority warns that canned commercial formula can expose infants to 13 mcg of BPA per kilogram of body weight, on a daily basis.

DAMAGED PROTEINS

The high-heat processing of all formulas (whether powdered or liquid) denatures proteins. This means that when exposed to high temperatures, the "3-D" molecular structure of proteins becomes flattened, and they lose their natural ability to function normally, potentially rendering them unfit for human consumption. When proteins are damaged in this way, they are more likely to be hard on the digestive system, allergenic, and can even be toxic.

MISSING FATS, WRONG FATS, IMBALANCED FATS, AND DAMAGED FATS

According to renowned pediatrician William Sears, M.D., a problem with the fat blends used in infant formulas is that they are completely lacking cholesterol. While cholesterol is inappropriately feared by many adults, babies *require* it because it supports cell membrane function, nerve transmission, and brain development. The fact that mom's milk contains plenty of cholesterol and also supplies nutrients that *increase* cholesterol's absorption underscores the importance of cholesterol in babies' diets.

Human Alternatives to Commercial Formula

From all mammalian milks considered, cow's milk has decidedly been the best base from which to make infant formula (commercial or homemade), with various additions to make it more nutritionally appropriate for human babies. The fact is, however, *human* milk is far better for human babies than is the milk of another species. We're just far more socially accepting of using a cow's "donor" udder milk rather than a human's donor breast milk. The United Nations Children's Fund (UNICEF) and the World Health Organization say that the best food for a baby who isn't fed his mother's milk is human milk from another healthy mother. The Human Milk-Banking Association of North America is a nonprofit association of donor human milk banks. Their website, www.hmbana.org, provides information on milk banking and how to contact a milk bank to donate milk or to order donor human milk.

Formula is also a poor source of important essential fatty acids like DHA and AA (or ARA). Those added to formulas are obtained from fermented fungus and algae, using a neurotoxic chemical solvent. They are easily damaged, often rendering them useless, from the heat, light, time, pressure, and chemicals to which they are exposed during processing, packaging, distribution, and storage.

Soy—A Troublemaker at All Ages

Promoted as a panacea of health, soy products have become popular to the point where they appear in every grocery store, from "health" foods to factory-farmed animal products. Soy derivatives are found in *nearly all* processed and packaged foods, used to make everything from veggie burgers and soy milk to snacks and cereals. Without even trying, the average American gets nearly 1 out of every 10 calories from soy alone—not many other single foods have such a high percentage of daily intake (except for corn and sugar)!

Soy is *not* the health food it is advertised to be. It is important to understand the very real health risks posed by soy consumption because it is actually a health hazard. In fact, below is just a partial list of the ill effects linked to soy—at any age. Studies have shown that soy can:

▸ Block thyroid function, and thus particular caution should be taken with babies who have congenital hypothyroidism

▸ Hinder protein breakdown

▸ Disrupt the endocrine system (glands such as pituitary and thyroid that control basic body functions)

▸ Be linked to an increased risk of cancer, particularly breast

▸ Irritate the digestive system, causing digestive distress

▸ Alter neurotransmitters, possibly leading to neurological and psychological disorders

Further, soy:

▸ Contains oxalates (most kidney stones are caused by high-oxalate foods)

▸ Increases the need for vitamin B12 because soy can block the ability of true B12 from being absorbed from other foods; B12 is critical to prevent anemia, serves red blood cells, supports proper nerve development, and aids in food digestion

▸ Is almost always genetically modified, unless organic or stated to be not genetically modified (non-GMO); GMO foods are exposed to more pesticides, and studies indicate they can lead to cancer, infertility, organ problems, and immune disruptions (For more on GMO, see page 149.)

▸ Blocks mineral absorption, reducing key minerals like iron, zinc, magnesium, copper, and calcium

▸ Contains excessive manganese (linked to brain damage in infants)

SOY IN INFANT FEEDING

In addition to general concerns about soy, there are specific concerns related to soy-based infant feeding. While the AAP states very few reasons to give soy formula to infants, statistics show 25 percent of formula-fed babies are given soy formula.

Severe GI effects from soy. The AAP reports, "Severe gastrointestinal reactions to soy protein formula have been described for greater than 30 years." Complications include severe bloody diarrhea, ulcerations, and acute and chronic inflammatory bowel disease.

Allergenic likelihood. Soy is one of the eight foods that cause 90 percent of food allergies. According to the National Institute of Allergy and Infectious Disease, U.S.

Department of Health and Human Services, soy allergies particularly affect infants. In fact, soy has up to fifteen different proteins that can cause allergic reactions, ranging from mild to life-threatening anaphylaxis.

Mineral deficiencies. As we discussed in chapter 2, infants around 6 months of age have a critical need for iron and zinc. Soy-based formula contains considerable amounts of phytates that markedly block the absorption of these (and other) minerals.

Soy is an even bigger no-no for preemies. The AAP clearly warns, "soy formulas are not recommended for preterm infants." This conclusion stems from studies showing that soy formula feeding could lead to the mineral deficiency–related disease osteopenia and other health complications.

Exceptions to the No-Soy Rule

Soy is not good for anyone, but it's particularly bad for pregnant and nursing mothers, infants, and children. The one exception to this rule is organic fermented soy—as in miso (soybean paste), natto (steamed and mashed soybeans), and tempeh (cooked soybean cake)—which can be incorporated in small amounts into a healthy diet. Vitamin K2 is found in high amounts in fermented natto. Tamari soy sauce, another form of fermented soy, is also safe to use sparingly. Remember that unless it's labeled "certified organic," assume soy is genetically modified, as it almost always is.

Reproductive development disruption. According to the National Institutes of Health, recent research has shown that soy's isoflavones (phyto-, or plant-based, estrogens that mimic human estrogen) can cause "adverse effects on development." Genistein (an isoflavone in soy) has been found to trigger reproductive abnormalities, including a rare form of uterine cancer. Women who were fed soy formula as babies have been shown to have more menstrual discomfort, cycle irregularities, and more uterine fibroids. But soy's effects on infant reproductive development are even more alarming.

Babies fed soy formula receive daily doses of phytoestrogens that are *ten times* higher than those found in typical Asian diets and 3,000 times more than found in mom's milk from mothers eating soy. The Weston A. Price Foundation reports that exclusively soy-fed babies have 13,000 to 22,000 times more serum estrogen compounds than do babies fed cow's milk formula. Extrapolating the data, these babies may be ingesting the daily estrogen equivalent of three to five birth control pills.

During development, baby boys normally have a dramatic increase in testosterone during their early months—some levels as high as an adult male! Soy's high amounts of estrogen have the potential to confuse characteristically male behaviors and normal physical development.

For girls, the AAP reports that puberty is starting earlier than ever before. Animal studies suggest that this might be related to overall exposure to soy, from phytoestrogens in soy formula to large quantities of soy in processed foods. Animals fed soy have shown effects such as "early onset of puberty in females and alterations in development of breast tissue," reports the National Institute of Environmental Health Sciences.

If Commercial Formula Is Your Only Option

Add cod liver oil. Make sure to add 1 teaspoon of high-quality cod liver oil or $1/2$ teaspoon fermented cod liver oil to it. And as soon as possible (4 months of age), introduce solid foods like egg yolk, liver, meat, and bone broths.

Add beneficial bacteria, too. Even if the formula you've selected has probiotics added, it is doubtful they've survived the processing and shelf life; therefore, additional supplementation is beneficial. We recommend $1/4$ teaspoon per day of bifidobacterium infantis powder either added to formula or directly provided on a moistened fingertip.

Super Nutrition Food Categorizations for 0 to 6 Months

Super POWER	PURE
Mom's milk	Homemade formula
OKAY	**CRAP**
Enriched formula	Commercial formula, especially soy

More bad ingredients. If the multiple serious risks of soy itself weren't enough, there are additional ingredients found in soy formula that are toxic for your baby, including corn syrup and sucrose, ten times the amount of manganese found in cow's milk formula (50 to 75 times that which is found in mom's milk), as well as high quantities of aluminum and fluoride.

Better Options Than Store-Bought Formulas

Both the AAP and the FDA discourage homemade formula because, *if done carelessly or incorrectly*, it can lead to potentially dangerous nutrient deficiencies, particularly if cow's milk or goat's milk alone is given. While we acknowledge the risk, we also know that correctly made homemade formula is *by far* the best alternative to mom's milk and a far more natural option than store-bought, commercial formula. This kind of formula is what you can feed your baby and feel good about, rather than wondering what bad things are in the powdered stuff.

It is critical to realize that, in making homemade formula, the FDA cautions "great care" is required and "safety should be a prime concern." If a scientifically based recipe

meeting all nutritional needs is not followed to the letter, potential problems could be "very serious and range from severe nutritional imbalances to unsafe products that can harm infants." However, don't let this discourage you. Considering the potential impurities and imbalances in store-bought formula, as we've mentioned, there are potentially more serious risks involved with commercial formula. We feel *you* are the best person to ensure your baby's safety and well-being, far better than any huge company that is more interested in taking your money than protecting and nourishing your child. Increasing numbers of parents are making homemade formula—resulting in many health benefits (over commercial formula) for their babies.

If you are unable to pay astute attention to making homemade formula, then we urge you *not* to do it, but rather enrich conventional formula (instructions appear on page 208). If, however, you are motivated and willing to learn, and will be cautious, careful, and fastidious in taking on this responsibility, then homemade formula will provide Super Nutrition for your baby, helping to ensure proper physical growth and cognitive development—which are both occurring so rapidly at this age.

Just like this mom in 1946, you do want to be relaxed when you feed your baby. They had the right idea, saying that "Mother is doubly relaxed and peaceful when," what she feeds her baby is prepared especially "for easy digestion" and contains the nutrients her baby needs. By using a digestible, nutritious, natural, wholesome homemade formula, you can rest easy when you hold your baby close to feed him.

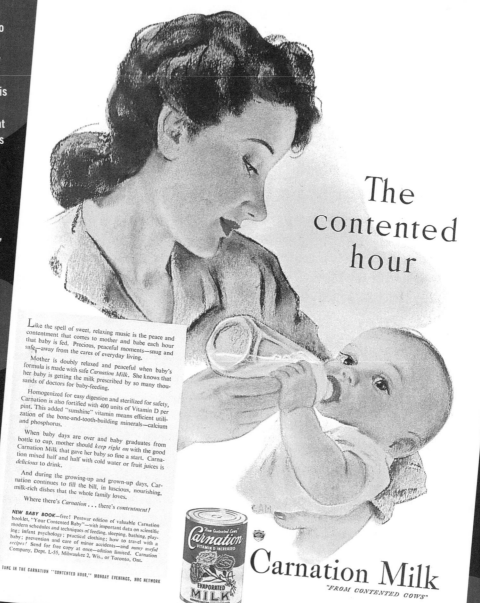

PRACTICAL FEEDING TIPS FOR NEWBORNS

When making homemade formula for your baby, you are taking steps to provide ultimate nourishment second only to mom's milk. The bottle-feeding experience can be improved, as well, by applying some of the following formula-feeding guidelines and practical considerations.

Close contact during feeding. Human contact is a critical part of feeding in infancy and is actually important for baby's health. Bottle or breast, your baby should be fed while being held close, cuddled, preferably with skin-to-skin contact as well as with eye contact and emotional interaction. This sense of security will ease any discomfort and provide reassurance, relaxation, and ease of mind so that your baby can focus on swallowing, digesting, and utilizing nutrients optimally.

On cue. Begin to prepare your baby's bottle when she shows the first signs of being ready to eat (wakefulness, alertness, rooting or sucking motions, or bringing hands to

Pattern	Second half of 6th month
Early AM	Milk / homemade formula
Mid-Morning	New choice
Mid-Day	Milk / homemade formula
Afternoon	Milk / homemade formula (before nap)
Evening	Already-introduced food
Nighttime	Milk / homemade formula (before bed)

mouth). It is especially important to heed very early hunger cues in a baby who is being bottle fed due to the additional preparation time (mixing, heating, and temperature checking) needed. Crying and agitation are *late* signals of hunger.

Warming Warnings

Never microwave your baby's formula. It damages the proteins and fats, and hot spots can develop. Also, avoid aluminum and Teflon-coated pans in your formula preparation as well as plastic containers for storage. Ideally, heat in glass, stainless steel, or ceramic. We recommend heating formula to body temperature (98.6°F or 37°C), which is what your baby will expect. Put a little on your wrist to test the formula prior to feeding—the right temperature is when you can't feel warmth or coolness.

How much to offer? There is no exact amount of formula necessarily recommended per feeding, but the standard "rule" for full-term babies is about 1 ounce (28 ml) per hour. Thus, if your baby sleeps 3 hours and wakes hungry, expect to feed him 3 ounces (90 ml); if he sleeps 2 hours, offer 2 ounces (60 ml). Just after birth, this amount may be a little less; and as he grows, your baby will take more. If he sucks the bottle dry, put an additional 1/2 ounce (14 ml) in the next bottle at the next feeding and keep increasing by 1/2 ounce (14 ml) until you reach a volume where he doesn't finish it all and a little remains. Always plan on wasting a little at the end of each feeding, as it is this final amount that clues you in to how much formula your baby needs. If he drinks it all, it wasn't enough. If some is left then he's had all he needs that feeding. Never force your baby to finish his bottle.

Bottle and nipple preparation. Before first use, wash bottles and nipples with soap and then boil for 5 minutes to reduce chemicals. For routine sterilization, either wash bottles and nipples in a dishwasher that reaches 180°F (82°C) or boil for 10 minutes.

Water matters. The American Dental Association supports not using fluorinated water for babies' formula "to reduce the risk of fluorosis." (For more information on the risks of fluoride, see page 71.) Well water should also be filtered and routinely tested for toxins and bacteria. Tap or municipal water also has "water treatment by-products" including chlorine and various chemicals like cancer-causing arsenic and perchlorate (rocket fuel). Chlorine and perchlorate (made from chlorine) further contribute to iodine deficiency and thus the mental decline of future generations. An ideal water to use is reverse osmosis–filtered water because it removes fluoride, chlorine, and other toxic materials from water.

Proceed with Caution

We strongly advise that in making homemade formula, you follow the recipes exactly as written. Do not make any substitutions, leave out any ingredients, or veer from the specific directions. Just as in the early days of commercial formula, when there are missing ingredients or inaccurate ratios, babies can become sick, and if nutrient needs are not properly met, malnutrition can lead to failure to thrive.

FORMULA RECIPES THAT PROVIDE OPTIMAL NOURISHMENT FOR GROWING BABIES

The three homemade formulas provided in this chapter are a cow's milk recipe, a goat's milk variation, and a meat/liver-derived recipe. The recipes were developed by (and are used with the permission of) members of the Weston A. Price Foundation (WAPF), including doctors, scientists, and other nutrition and traditional-foods experts, such as Mary Enig, Ph.D.; they provide the healthiest ingredients for your baby when it comes to formula.

Breast Milk and Homemade Formulas Nutrient Comparison Chart

The Weston A. Price Foundation (WAPF) has compiled a nutrient-comparison chart, reprinted here with permission, for their three formula recipes and mom's milk. WAPF notes, "These nutrient comparison tables were derived from standard food nutrient tables and do not take into account the wide variation in nutrient levels that can occur in both human and animal milk, depending on diet and environment." For a deeper comparison of mom's milk, cow's milk formula, goat's milk formula, and meat-based formula, visit www.westonaprice.org. Select "order materials" and choose the "Breast Milk/Formula Flier." It is based on 36 ounces (1 L).

Mom to Mom / You can skim off cream that rises to the top of your raw milk and use the remaining "skimmed" milk to make whey. (See the recipe for Homemade Whey in this chapter or in chapter 2.) Do not use half-and-half or powdered whey. Whey can be made from clabbered (soured) raw milk, or it can be made from plain, organic yogurt from the store.

In order to make your own formula, you'll need to do some legwork to get all the ingredients, but that's the hardest part. (Note: See Resources on page 218 for where to purchase some of these ingredients.) Once you've gotten everything and made formula once, it gets easier. Your efforts are well worth it and will provide your baby with a natural, real-food–based formula that is more protective, more nourishing, and less harmful and risky than mass-produced, highly processed, commercial formula. WAPF acknowledges that parents who invest the time "will be well rewarded with the joys of conferring robust good health on their children."

Breast Milk and Homemade Formulas Nutrient Comparision Chart

Nutrient	Breast Milk	Cow's Milk Formula	Goat's Milk Formula	Liver-Based Formula
Calories	766	856	890	682
Protein	11.3 g	18 g	18 g	15 g
Carbohydrates	76 g	79 g	77 g	69 g
Total fat	48 g	52 g	54 g	36 g
Saturated fat	22 g	28 g	30 g	16 g
Monounsaturated fat	18 g	16 g	16 g	12 g
Polyunsaturated fat	5.5 g	5.6 g	5.7 g	5.6 g
Omega-3 fatty acids	0.58 g	1.3 g	1.2 g	1.0 g
Omega-6 fatty acids	4.4 g	4.2 g	4.4 g	4.5 g
Cholesterol	153 mg	137 mg	166 mg	227 mg
Vitamin A*	946 IU	5,000 IU	5,000 IU	20,000 IU
Thiamin-B1	0.15 mg	1.05 mg	1.1 mg	0.19 mg
Riboflavin-B2	0.4 mg	1.2 mg	1.2 mg	1.9 mg
Niacin-B3	1.9 mg	2.5 mg	4.4 mg	14.2 mg
Vitamin B6	0.12 mg	0.51 mg	0.60 mg	0.65 mg
Vitamin B12	0.5 mcg	1.9 mcg	2.8 mcg	39 mcg
Folate	57 mcg	236 mcg	284 mcg	159 mcg
Vitamin C	55 mg	57 mg	59 mg	62 mg

Nutrient	Breast Milk	Cow's Milk Formula	Goat's Milk Formula	Liver-Based Formula
Vitamin D	480 IU	450 IU	525 IU	460 IU
Vitamin E**	9.9 mg	6.2 mg	4.7 mg	4.9 mg
Calcium	355 mg	532 mg	548 mg	NA***
Copper	0.57 mg	0.38 mg	0.58 mg	1.9 mg
Iron	0.33 mg	1.4 mg	2.2 mg	5.4 mg
Magnesium	37.4 mg	91.3 mg	96.1 mg	34.5 mg
Manganese	0.29 mg	0.034 mg	0.12 mg	0.24 mg
Phosphorus	151 mg	616 mg	729 mg	344 mg
Potassium	560 mg	949 mg	1228 mg	750 mg
Selenium	18.8 mcg	15.4 mcg	18.7 mcg	31.1 mcg
Sodium	186 mg	308 mg	320 mg	NA***
Zinc	1.9 mg	2.8 mg	2.7 mg	2.5 mg

*Vitamin A levels in human milk will depend on the diet of the mother. Nursing mothers eating vitamin A–rich foods such as cod liver oil will have much higher levels of vitamin A in their milk. Commercial formulas contain about 2,400 IU vitamin A per 800 calories.

**Vitamin E values are derived from commercial vegetable oils. The vitamin E levels for homemade formulas will be higher if good-quality, expeller-expressed oils are used.

***Calcium and sodium values for homemade broth are not available.

Mom to Mom / Though formula should be made fresh daily, freezing it in individual 4- to 9-ounce (120 to 250 ml) serving sizes is fine. It may be stored in the freezer for 2 to 3 months. After defrosting, add ¼ teaspoon of probiotics per day. Be aware that after defrosting, the cream's consistency may change. If frozen, warm formula by setting jars in warm water to thaw.

The following recipes are printed verbatim from the Weston A. Price Foundation. Do not vary *at all* from these recipes.

Raw Milk Baby Formula

Our milk-based formula takes account of the fact that human milk is richer in whey, lactose, vitamin C, niacin, and long-chain polyunsaturated fatty acids compared to cow's milk but is leaner in casein (milk protein). The addition of gelatin to cow's milk formula will make it more digestible for the infant. Use only truly expeller-expressed oils in the formula recipes; otherwise they may lack vitamin E.

The ideal milk for baby, if he cannot be breast-fed, is clean, whole raw milk from old-fashioned cows, certified free of disease, that feed on green pasture. For sources of good-quality milk, see www.realmilk.com or contact a local chapter of the Weston A. Price Foundation.

If the only choice available to you is commercial milk, choose whole milk, preferably organic and unhomogenized, and culture it with a piima or kefir culture to restore enzymes. (See Sources of Ingredients and Supplies for Homemade Formula, page 213.)

Culturing milk is usually as simple as following the kefir culture directions and typically includes mixing a powder packet with the instructed amount of milk and allowing the mixture to ferment on your counter at room temperature for about 24 hours.

According to WAPF, however, if you don't have access to raw, clean, grass-fed milk, then the meat-based formula (page 206) would be your best alternative.

1 ⅞ cups (440 ml) filtered water

2 teaspoons gelatin

4 tablespoons (52 g) lactose

2 teaspoons virgin coconut oil

¼ teaspoon high-vitamin butter oil (optional, but highly recommended)

2 cups (475 ml) whole, raw milk from organic, grass-fed Jersey cows

¼ cup (60 ml) liquid whey (Do NOT use powdered whey from the store or whey from making cheese.) (See the recipe for Homemade Whey from Store-Bought Dairy, page 207.)

¼ teaspoon bifidobacterium powder

2 tablespoons (28 ml) good-quality raw or pasteurized cream (not ultrapasteurized) (Use 4 tablespoons [60 ml] if the milk is from Holstein cows.)

½ teaspoon unflavored, fermented cod liver oil ("Salty cod" is the one you want, but plain or antioxidant-free cod liver oil can alternatively be used.)

1 teaspoon expeller sunflower oil

1 teaspoon organic, extra-virgin olive oil (in a dark bottle)

2 teaspoons Frontier nutritional yeast flakes

¼ teaspoon acerola powder

Fill a 2-cup (475 ml) glass measuring cup with the filtered water and remove 2 tablespoons (28 ml) (this will give you 1⅞ cups ([440 ml] water). Pour about half the water into a (nonaluminum, preferably stainless steel) saucepan and put over medium heat.

Add the gelatin and lactose and let dissolve, stirring occasionally. Once dissolved, remove the saucepan from the heat and add the rest of the water to cool it slightly.

Stir in the coconut oil and butter oil, if using, until melted.

Put the remaining ingredients in a glass blender. Add the water mixture and blend for about 3 seconds until everything is combined.

Place the formula in very clean glass bottles or a glass jar and refrigerate.

Before giving to baby, warm a glass bottle in a pan of hot water or a bottle warmer. (Never heat formula in a microwave oven!)

Yield: 36 ounces (1 L)

Why Fresh, Raw Milk?

Using raw, grass-fed, unpasteurized milk from a trusted, clean dairy, with a few tweaks necessary to make it optimally nutritious for your baby, results in an infant formula that is much closer to mom's milk than anything else could possibly be. As we discussed in chapter 1, being raw means that the milk is living. And similar to human milk—which is also fed raw to babies—it retains various live constituents needed for optimal growth, development, and immunity. Destroyed by pasteurization and homogenization, these factors are unique to raw milk (human, cow, and goat) and are critical to your baby's health.

Pasteurizing milk destroys and damages nutritious proteins, vitamins, minerals, and immune-bolstering components found in fresh milk. This can result in an immune response to the pasteurized milk—kicking off allergies, asthma, or autoimmune conditions as well as taxing enzymes, digestion, energy, and nutrient stores. Fresh, raw milk, however, digests itself, rather than depleting nutrient and enzyme stores to digest it. *Raw* milk supplies nutrient-rich and immune-boosting factors that are effortlessly assimilated. Visit www.realmilk.com for more important information.

Notes

- Mixed formula ideally should be made daily and can last 24 hours in the refrigerator. It can be left at room temperature for a few hours.
- See Resources, page 218, for ingredients and supplies for homemade formula.

Variation: Goat's Milk Formula

For some infants, the goat's milk protein is easier to digest than that found in cow's milk. WAPF instructs: Although goat milk is rich in fat, it must be used with caution in infant feeding as it lacks folic acid and is low in vitamin B12, both of which are essential to the growth and development of the infant. Inclusion of nutritional yeast to provide folic acid is essential.

To compensate for low levels of vitamin B12, if preparing the Milk-Based Formula (above) with goat's milk, add 2 teaspoons organic raw chicken liver, frozen for 14 days, finely grated to the batch of formula. Be sure to begin egg-yolk feeding at 4 months.

Note

- Mixed formula ideally should be made daily and can last 24 hours in the refrigerator. It can be left at room temperature for a few hours.

Liver-Based Formula

The following recipe is for meat-based formula, which is considered hypoallergenic as it does not contain milk proteins from goats or cows.

Our liver-based formula also mimics the nutrient profile of mother's milk. It is extremely important to include coconut oil in this formula, as it is the only ingredient that provides the special medium-chain saturated fats found in mother's milk. As with the milk-based formula, all oils should be truly expeller expressed.

2 ounces (55 g) organic liver, cut into small pieces

3³/₄ cups (887 ml) homemade beef or chicken broth (page 56)

5 tablespoons (65 g) lactose

¹/₄ teaspoon bifidobacterium infantis powder

¹/₄ cup (60 ml) homemade liquid whey (See recipe for Homemade Whey from Store-Bought Dairy, page 207)

1 tablespoon (14 g) coconut oil

¹/₂ teaspoon unflavored high-vitamin or high-vitamin fermented cod liver oil, or 1 teaspoon regular cod liver oil (Use only recommended brands.)

1 teaspoon unrefined sunflower oil

2 teaspoons extra-virgin olive oil (in a dark bottle)

¼ teaspoon acerola powder

Simmer the liver gently in the broth until the meat is cooked through.

Liquefy using a handheld blender or in a food processor.

When the liver broth has cooled, stir in the remaining ingredients. Store in a very clean glass or stainless steel container in the refrigerator.

To serve, stir the formula well and pour 6 to 8 ounces (175 to 235 ml) in a very clean glass bottle. Attach a clean nipple and set in a pan of simmering water until the formula is warm but not hot to the touch. Shake well and feed to baby. (Never heat formula in a microwave oven!)

Notes

- Lactose, coconut oil, unrefined sunflower oil, extra-virgin olive oil, and acerola powder are available from Radiant Life (see Resources, page 218). Refer to Resources for other ingredients and supplies to make this formula.
- Beef or lamb liver are the best early options. When your baby is older than 6 months, chicken or buffalo liver can be substituted.
- Mixed formula should be kept about 24 hours in the refrigerator, ideally made daily. It can be left at room temperature for a few hours.

Yield: About 36 ounces (1 L)

Homemade Whey from Store-Bought Dairy

Homemade whey is easy to make from good-quality plain yogurt or from raw or cultured milk. See other Whey recipes, page 64 or use this recipe from the excellent nutritional and culinary resource Nourishing Traditions *by Sally Fallon.*

You will need a large strainer that rests over a bowl.

If you are using yogurt, place 2 quarts (1.9 L) in the strainer lined with a tea towel. Cover with a plate and leave at room temperature overnight. The whey will drip out into the bowl. Place whey in clean glass jars and store in the refrigerator.

If you are using raw or cultured milk, place 2 quarts (1.9 L) of the milk in a glass container and leave at room temperature for 2 to 4 days until the milk separates into curds and whey. Pour into the strainer lined with a tea towel and cover with a plate. Leave at room temperature overnight. The whey will drip out into the bowl. Store in clean glass jars in the refrigerator.

Yield: About 5 cups (1 L)

- See Resources, page 218, for ingredients and supplies for homemade whey.

"Enriched" Commercial, Organic, Cow's Milk Formula

If it's not possible to make any of the formulas (exactly as stated) in the previous recipes, your next best option is to "improve" commercial formula by adding a few key ingredients that will make it more digestible and more nutritious for your baby. This formula can also be used as a stopgap in emergencies or when the ingredients for homemade formula are unavailable. WAPF has formulated this recipe, reprinted with permission, for improving upon commercial formula.

1 cup (235 ml) milk-based powdered formula*

3⁵⁄₈ cups (29 ounces, or 835 ml) filtered water

1 large egg yolk from an organic egg

¹⁄₂ teaspoon unflavored high-vitamin or high-vitamin fermented cod liver oil, or 1 teaspoon regular cod liver oil (Use only recommended brands of cod liver oil, as noted in Resources.)

Place all ingredients in a blender or food processor and blend thoroughly. Store in a very clean glass jar in the refrigerator.

To serve, put 6 to 8 ounces (175 to 235 ml) of formula in a clean glass bottle. Attach a clean nipple to the bottle and set in a pan of simmering water until the formula is warm but not hot to the touch. Gently shake well and feed to baby. (Never heat formula in a microwave oven!)

Yield: About 35 ounces (1 L)

Notes

- Mixed formula should ideally be made daily and can last 24 hours in the refrigerator. It can be left at room temperature for a few hours.
- You can opt to first boil the egg as descried on pg 55 for 3½ minutes (especially if you have low quality eggs).

*The best choice for commercial formula today seems to be Baby's Only Organic Dairy Formula. It contains iron and better ingredients than any of the other commercial formulas. It is also the only brand on the market at this time without damaged essential fatty acids DHA and ARA, which can be inflammatory and lead to oxidative stress. If Baby's Only Organic Dairy Formula is not available, we recommend an organic cow's milk formula with certain key additions.

Afterword

"Life in all its fullness is Mother Nature obeyed."

—WESTON A. PRICE, D.D.S.

At two-years-old, you've surely got an adorable little busy body. As she continues to rapidly learn and grow, her exploration of the world might now include more playdates with friends, outings, and even possibly preschool next year. While these new experiences will bring challenges of their own, we hope the suggestions and information gained from this book will have helped you to create a strong and secure foundation. Continue to take pride in every small step forward you take to provide your baby with Super Nutrition, and know that your efforts are well worth it.

With the nutritional knowledge and commitment you now have, you can continue to positively influence your child's health destiny, steering her toward optimal health and the ability to live a full and rich life.

Appendix

Food Introduction Timeline

This timeline includes Super POWER and PURE foods that may or may not have been discussed in previous chapters. At each age, continue offering foods from the previous stages. With this excellent foundation, mixing in some OKAY foods, as needed, is acceptable. We of course caution you to avoid CRAP foods for as long as possible.

0 to 4 months	Mom's milk, homemade formula, and probiotics in special cases*; nursing moms: eat Super POWER foods and supplement with vitamin D, cod liver oil, 5-MTHF, B12 and probiotics.
4 to 6 months	Egg yolk, cod liver oil, and liver in special cases**
6 months	Egg yolk, grated frozen liver, Souper Stock, meats in soups, and unpasteurized sauerkraut juice in special cases*** (see chapter 2)
6.5 months	Avocado, banana, cooked sweet potato (lacto-fermented preferred), carrots cooked in soup with marrow or ghee, and kidneys and other organ meats
7 months	Cooked apples and pears, poultry, fish roe, marrow, other meats, lacto-fermented veggies, and tropical fruits
8 months	Cumin, garlic, olive oil, coconut milk and coconut kefir, sea salt, pork (bacon, ham, sausage), schmaltz and lard, zucchini, parsnips, cooked peaches, nectarines, and cherries

9 months	Raw yogurt, raw butter, raw cheese, raw puréed fruits, oily fish, passion fruit, pomegranate, guava, Goji berries, pineapple, cooked onion, mulberries, cooked strawberries, blackberries, blueberries, and raspberries, gelatin jigglers, olives, and unpasteurized pickles
10 months	Coconut water, beets, filtered water, more herbs and spices, beet kvass, and well-steamed leafy greens (spinach, kale)
11 months	Fish stocks and stews and deep-sea wild-caught fish
12 to 15 months	Whole eggs, honey (raw, unheated, unfiltered), tomato, white potato, eggplant, peppers, citrus fruits (lemon, lime, grapefruit, orange, and tangerine), seasonings (paprika), tomatillos, pimentos, blackstrap molasses, maple syrup, other natural sweeteners in extremely small quantities, arrowroot starch, raw dairy milk, barley water, soaked nuts, liverwurst, cinnamon, vanilla, whole plant stevia, turnips, homemade juice, well-cooked leafy greens (Swiss chard, collard, beet, and mustard greens), celery, radishes, beets, uncooked berries, and cranberries
15 to 18 months	Nuts (preferably soaked and dried, including almonds, hazelnuts, walnuts, pecans, pistachios, macadamia nuts, and cashews) and nut butters, soaked brown rice, kombucha, apple cider, ginger ale, homemade orangina, raw veggies (tender greens like butterleaf, carrots, cucumbers), carob (limited) and sprouted seeds
18 to 21 months	Properly prepared gluten-free grains, raw greens (all of the above except kale and collard greens still cooked); higher-fiber raw veggies; and pasteurized cheese (on occasion, only if raw is not available)
21 to 24 months	Properly prepared gluten grains, properly prepared legumes (peanuts, green beans, and chickpeas) and shellfish (oysters, sea cucumber, clams, scallops, mussels, lobster, sea urchins, and shrimp)
2 years +	Rarely: pasteurized dairy (preferably plain, cultured, whole, grass-fed, organic, nonhomogenized), dried fruit, fermented soy (natto, miso, tempeh), unsoaked nuts, tea, seeds not sprouted, nitrite/nitrate-free organic lunch meat, and peanut butter

* If born by C-section or mom or baby received antibiotics or steroids, start probiotic supplements right after birth.

** Start very-first foods at 4 months for babies fed commercial formula, assuming early signs of being ready to eat are met. (Never start first foods before 4 months.) It is important to start liver early when there is iron deficiency, failure to thrive, formula issues, and with vegetarian mothers.

*** When there are digestive issues like reflux/spitting up or a personal or family history of 3Cs or digestion issues

Recommended Reading and Documentaries

Don't Stop Here. The following are books, DVDs, and websites that we have referenced throughout the book or that have positively impacted our views and understanding of food. While these are excellent sources of nutritional information, they aren't the only resources available. We provide them as a place to start, hoping that you will continue to build upon your solid foundation of traditional-foods knowledge. We encourage you to seek out even more information to support your crusade for better health for your family.

TRADITIONAL FOODS AND FOOD PREPARATION

- *Nourishing Traditions*, Sally Fallon
- *Healing Our Children*, Ramiel Nagel
- *The Whole Beast; Nose to Tail Eating*, Fergus Henderson
- *The Grassfed Gourmet*, Shannon Hayes
- *Pasture Perfect*, Jo Robinson
- *Wild Fermentation*, Sandor Ellix Katz
- *Truly Cultured*, Nancy Lee Bentley
- *Recipes for the Specific Carbohydrate Diet*, Raman Prasad

- *Eat Fat Lose Fat*, Dr. Mary Enig, Ph.D., and Sally Fallon

- *Wholesome Home Cooking—Preparing Nutrient-Dense Foods*, Katie L. Stoltzfus

- *The Whole Soy Story*, Kaayla T. Daniel, Ph.D.

- *Trick and Treat: How "Healthy Eating" Is Making Us Ill*, Dr. Barry Groves

- *Traditional Foods Are Your Best Medicine*, Ronald F. Schmid, N.D.

3C CONDITIONS AND CHILDREN'S HEALTH

- *Healing and Preventing Autism*, Jenny McCarthy and Dr. Jerry Kartzinel

- *Gut and Psychology Syndrome*, Natasha Campbell-McBride, M.D., MMedSci.

- *The NDD™ Book*, William Sears

- *Healing the New Childhood Epidemics*, Kenneth Bock, M.D.

- *Digestive Wellness for Children*, Elizabeth Lipski, Ph.D., C.C.N.

- *The Puzzle of Autism*, Dr. Amy Yasko and Dr. Garry Gordon

- *Compromised Generation: The Epidemic of Chronic Illness in America's Children*, Beth Lambert

- *Nourishing Hope for Autism*, Julie Matthews

SUGAR ADDICTION

- *Little Sugar Addicts*, Kathleen DesMaisons, Ph.D.

- *The Anatomy of a Food Addiction*, Anne Katherine

- *Lick the Sugar Habit*, Nancy Appleton, Ph.D.

- *Sugar Blues*, William F. Duffy

- *Suicide by Sugar*, Nancy Appleton, Ph.D.

- *The Hidden Addiction and How to Get Free*, Janice Keller Phelps, M.D., and Alan Nourse, M.D.

- *Sugar . . . Stop the Addiction*, Kelly Genzlinger, C.N.C.

GENERAL AND CHILDREN'S NUTRITION AND FOOD-RELATED HEALTH

- *The Truth about Children's Health: The Comprenhensive Guide to Understanding, Preventing, and Reversing Disease*, Robert Bernardini, M.S.

- *An Encyclopedia of Natural Healing for Children and Infants*, Mary Bove, N.D.

- *Our Children's Health: America's Kids in Nutritional Crisis and What We Can Do to Help Them*, Bonnie C. Minsky

- *Iodine: Why We Need It; Why We Can't Live Without It*, David Brownstein, M.D.

- *Salt Your Way to Health*, David Brownstein, M.D.

- *The Guide to a Gluten-Free Diet*, David Brownstein, M.D., and Sheryl Shenefelt, C.N.

- *The Soy Deception*, David Brownstein, M.D., and Sheryl Shenefelt, C.N.

- *Real Food for Mother and Baby*, Nina Planck

- *Could It Be B12?*, Sally M. Pacholok, R.N., Jeffrey J. Stuart, D.O.

- *Good Calories, Bad Calories*, Gary Taubes

- *The Vegetarian Myth*, Lierre Keith

- *Healthy 4 Life Dietary Guidelines*, The Weston A. Price Foundation

- *Vitamin K2 and the Calcium Paradox*, Kate Rheaume-Bleue, BSc., N.D.

FRESH, RAW MILK

- *The Untold Story of Milk*, Dr. Ronald F. Schmid, N.D.

- *The Raw Truth about Milk*, William Campbell Douglass II, M.D.

- *Milk Diet as a Remedy for Chronic Disease*, Charles Sanford Porter, M.D.

- *Raw Milk Revolution: The Emerging Battle over America's Food Rights*, David E. Gumpert

- *Nature's Healing Gift* (an eBook of personal raw milk testimonials), compiled by Laura Kozicki—http://www.realmilk.com/natureshealinggift.html

- *Pottenger's Cats*, Francis Marion Pottenger, Jr., M.D.

ATTACHMENT PARENTING AND BABY CARE

- *The Attachment Parenting Book*, William Sears, M.D., and Martha Sears, R.N.

- *Continuum Concept*, Jean Liedloff

- *The Baby Bond*, Dr. Linda Folden Palmer

- *The Fussy Baby Book*, William Sears, M.D., and Martha Sears, R.N.

THE TRUTH ABOUT FATS

- *Know Your Fats*, Mary G. Enig, Ph.D.

- *The Cholesterol Myths*, Uffe Ravnskov

- *The Great Cholesterol Con*, Anthony Colpo

- *Stop Worrying about Cholesterol! Better Ways to Avoid a Heart Attack and Get Healthy*, Richard E. Tapert, D.O.

- *The Queen of Fats*, Susan Allport

- *The Coconut Oil Miracle*, Bruce Fife

- *The Palm Oil Miracle*, Bruce Fife

VACCINE AWARENESS

- *The Sanctity of Human Blood: Vaccination Is Not Immunization*, Tim O'Shea

- *What Your Doctor May NOT Tell You About Children's Vaccinations*, Stephanie Cave, M.D.

- *The Vaccine Book: Making the Right Decision for Your Child*, Robert W. Sears, M.D.

- *Evidence of Harm*, David Kirby

- *A Shot in the Dark*, Harrison L. Coulter and Barbara Loe Fisher

- *Callous Disregard*, Dr. Andrew J. Wakefield

BREAST-FEEDING

- *The Breastfeeding Book*, William Sears, M.D., and Martha Sears, R.N.

- *The Womanly Art of Breastfeeding*, La Leche League International

- *Breastfeeding: Biocultural Perspectives*, Patricia Stuart-Macadam and Katherine A. Dettwyler

- *Breastfeeding a Toddler: Why on Earth?*, J. Jack Newman, M.D.

- *Mothering Your Nursing Toddler*, Norma J. Bumgarner

- *The Nursing Mother's Guide to Weaning*, Kathleen Huggins and Linda Ziedrich

Sources of Ingredients, Instructions, and Supplies for Homemade Formula

- http://www.radiantlifecatalog.com/product/HOMEMADE-BABY-FORMULA-INGREDIENTS/superfoods-supplements

COD LIVER OIL—RECOMMENDED BRANDS

- http://www.westonaprice.org/cod-liver-oil/

TO FIND A TRUSTED SOURCE OF RAW MILK NEAR YOU

- http://www.realmilk.com/where.html.

VIDEO ON HOW TO MAKE HYPOALLERGENIC BABY FORMULA

- http://www.thehealthyhomeeconomist.com/2010/09/video-hypoallergenic-baby-formula/

RESOURCE PAGE FOR HOMEMADE FORMULA

- http://www.westonaprice.org/childrens-health/recipes-for-homemade-baby-formula.html

HOMEMADE FORMULA TESTIMONIALS

- http://www.westonaprice.org/childrens-health/1307.html

THE RECIPES

- http://www.realmilk.com/formularecipes.html#chart

HOMEMADE FORMULA FAQS

- For answers to frequently asked questions about milk-based formula, visit http://www.westonaprice.org/faq/faq-homemade-baby-formula

HOMEMADE FORMULA (AMONG OTHER THINGS) PARENT GROUP

- Also, talk to other parents about their tips and tricks for homemade formula:

- A new Weston A. Price Healthy Babies Yahoo Group has been formed. Subjects will include preconception diets, pregnancy diets, breast-feeding, health issues, and homemade formula. Anyone is welcome. To register, go to http://healthgroups.yahoo.com/group.newwaphb/

KEFIR STARTER

- http://www.thehealthyhomeeconomist.com/resources/#starters

- http://www.bodyecology.com, G.E.M. Cultures, 1-800-511-2660

YEAST

- www.Iherb.com

RAW CREAM

- Order sources found in the Weston A. Price Shopping Guide at www.westonaprice.org

DOCUMENTARIES

- *InGREEDients*—www.ingreedientsmovie.com

- *Sweet Suicide*—http://nancyappleton.com/store/

- *Two Angry Moms*—http://www.angrymoms.org

- *The Oiling of America: How the Vegetable Industry Demonized Nutritious Animal Fats and Destroyed the American Food Supply*, DVD, Sally Fallon Morell, Phone (202) 363-4394 to order, Find on amazon.com, Watch: http://www.youtube.com/watch?v=N_O46Bml5JU

- *Nourishing Traditional Diets*: The Key to Vibrant Health, DVD, Sally Fallon Morell http://www.amazon.com

- *The Price Pottenger Story* (found at www.ppnf.org)

- *Fresh*—http://www.freshthemovie.com/

- *Healing Autism*, Kenneth Bock's DVD—http://www.healingautismdvd.com/

- PowerPoint presentation on Real Milk: http://www.realmilk.com/ppt/index.html

- *King Corn*—http://www.kingcorn.net/

- *What's On Your Plate?*—http://www.whatsonyourplateproject.org/

- *Food, Inc.*—http://www.foodincmovie.com/

- *In Search of the Perfect Human Diet*—http://www.perfecthumandiet.us

Resources

For guidelines that support traditional foods and Super Nutrition, see the Healthy 4 Life Guidelines from the Weston A. Price Foundation, as opposed to the USDA MyPlate, MyPyramid, and Food Pyramid dietary guidelines that support the food industry and improper eating.

- http://www.westonaprice.org—Select "Order Materials" on the right. Scroll down to "Healthy 4 Life Book" ($10). Further, for a shopping guide that organized grocery store and health food store items into quality rankings, order the WAPF Shopping Guide. This important guide will list brands and rank them as to their quality and value, from sauerkraut to yogurt and in between.

- http://www.westonaprice.org—Select "Order Materials" on the right. Scroll down to "Shopping Guide" ($1).

ONLINE INFORMATION AND RESOURCES

Traditional Foods and Real-Food Baby Feeding

- www.westonprice.org—a comprehensive and amazingly abundant resource on traditional foods and nutrition related to optimal health and disease prevention

- www.ninaplanck.com—author of Real Food for Mother and Baby, informative site on "real food" for real people living real lives

- www.westonaprice.org/childrens-health/feeding-babies—more information on nursing and baby feeding

- http://community.westonaprice.org/—discuss with a like-minded group living the traditional-foods lifestyle

- http://chriskregger.com—excellent blog on the truth about nutrition, food, and health

- www.westonaprice.org/soy-alert—for more about the actual effects of soy on health

- www.jamieoliver.com—revolutionary chef trying to change health by changing food, starting with children and school lunches

3C Conditions and Children's Health

- www.epidemicanswers.org—a wonderful site outlining information on many 3C conditions

- http://nourishinghope.com—website of author Julie Matthews, discussing dietary treatment for autism

- www.epidemicanswers.org—resources and information relating to common 3C conditions, including autism

- www.dramyyasko.com—information on the biochemical problems related to the 3Cs, detoxification and methylation pathway information, genetic testing, and more!

- www.healingthewholechild.com—Dr. Erlich's informative site—providing information, articles, and updates for Protective Nutrition

- www.nourishmd.com—informative articles and advice on "real-life" applications of healthy and traditional foods

- www.foodtherapeutics.com—Kelly Genzlinger's site discussing healthy eating guidelines and principles, favorite products, recommended reading, and more

Sugar and Health

- www.nancyappleton.com—pioneering whistle-blower on the dangers of dietary sugars

- www.hookedonjuice.com—for more information about the true risks of juice consumption

Vaccine and Antibiotic Information

- www.cdc.gov/vaccines/vac-gen/additives.htm—list of all vaccines and their ingredients

- www.nvic.org—vaccine rights advocacy and information

- www.toomanytoosoon.com—Dr. Bock's site on vaccines

- www.saveantibiotics.org—takes a scientific look at factory farming and the use of drugs in farming

Baby Care and Breastfeeding

- www.askdrsears.com—baby care, feeding, and parenting advice and a wealth of parenting, breast-feeding, and nutritional parenting information

- www.bloomsbabystuff.com—BabyRest nursing support pillow

Real Milk Information

- www.raw-milk-facts.com—information about raw, fresh milk

- www.realmilk.com—fresh milk info

- www.realmilk.com/raw.html—fresh milk info

- http://www.mercola.com/2004/apr/24/raw_milk.htm—fresh milk info

- http://www.usatoday.com/news/nation/tables/2006-08-06-raw-milk.htm—listing of which states allow raw milk sales

GMO Effects and Activism

- www.responsibletechnology.org—information and activism for GMO awareness

- www.responsibletechnology.org/blog/1412—Dangerous Toxins from Genetically Modified Plants Found in Women and Fetuses, article by Jeffrey Smith

Sources for Food, Supplements, Ingredients, Books, Equipment and More!

FOOD AND SUPPLEMENTS

- www.pureindianfoods.com—a great source of grass-fed ghee

- www.uswellnessmeats.com—liverwurst, liver, beef stock, grass-fed meat, organs, and bones

- www.vitalchoice.com—fish roe and high-quality fish

- www.livesuperfoods.com—fish roe and high-quality fish

- http://blog.grasslandbeef.com/super-nutrition-for-babies-0/—Super Nutrition for Babies specific selections from US Wellness Meats

- www.greenpasture.org—fermented cod liver oil and high-vitamin butter oil

- www.wateroz.com—Water of Life and mineral water supplements (consult a holistic practitioner)

- www.jcrowsmarketplace.com—Lugol's solution (iodine)

FOOD AND EQUIPMENT

- www.radiantlifecatalog.com—many items, including dehydrators, juicers, grain mills, pickling crocks, bath and shower water-filter systems, stainless children's dishes, stainless ice-cube trays, gelatin, arrowroot powder, crystal ball bath dechlorinator, EvenFlo glass bottles, Bariani olive oil, VioLiv glassware, and Nourishing Superfood Kit for Homemade Baby Formula

- www.thehappyherbalist.com—kombucha kits and more!

- www.amazon.com—source of some ingredients for homemade formula and for dolomite powder (you must purchase U.S. Pharmacopoeia (USP) dolomite, to avoid lead)

EQUIPMENT, BOOKS, AND MORE

- www.ppnf.org—provides many books on traditional foods, holistic health, and some products

- www.bambuhome.com—stainless steel cocktail spoons and bamboo spoons

- www.reuseit.com—sustainable, responsible storage containers and more

- www.laptoplunches.com—source of Bento box lunch systems for ease of taking food with you

- www.freshbaby.com—ice cube trays with plastic covers, BPA free and phthalate free

- www.krautpounder.com/—a hand-carved wooden tool that fits in mason jars to facilitate making your own lacto-fermented condiments

- www.organicbaby-yes.com—organic baby products

- www.babybullet.com—a useful tool in making baby food

- www.lalecheleague.org—1-800-LALECHE—breast-feeding support and information

COD LIVER OIL RECOMMENDATIONS

Sources (from the Weston A. Price Foundation):

Best: High-Vitamin Fermented Cod Liver Oil (CLO)

- Green Pasture Products: Blue Ice CLO (402) 858-4818, greenpasture.org

- Dr. Ron's Ultra-Pure: Blue Ice High-Vitamin Fermented CLO, (877) 472-8701, drrons.com

- Radiant Life: Blue Ice High-Vitamin Fermented CLO and Premier High-Vitamin CLO, (888) 593-8333, 4radiantlife.com

- Azure Standard: Blue Ice High-Vitamin Fermented CLO, (541) 467-2230, azurestandard.com

- Natural Health Advocates: Blue Ice High-Vitamin Fermented CLO, 888-257-8775, building-health.com/

- See http://www.westonaprice.org/cod-liver-oil/fclo-from-chapter-leaders.html our list local chapter leaders and members who sell fermented cod liver oil.

Good: Cod liver oil—tested free of heavy metals and other contaminants (available in stores)

- Carlson's

- Nordic Naturals

- Seroyal

- NOW double strength

- Sonne's

- Twin Labs

RESOURCES TO HELP YOU *FIND* HEALTHY, NOURISHING FOOD NEAR YOU

- Find a produce-providing, local, seasonal CSA near you—http://www.localharvest.org

- Find your local WAPF chapter—http://www.westonaprice.org/local-chapters/find-a-local-chapter—your local chapter will help with pastured animal foods, CSAs, and fresh, raw dairy

- Find fresh milk near you: http://www.realmilk.com/where1.html

- WAPF Shopping Guide—which will help you navigate the grocery store and find recommended brands—http://www.westonaprice.org (select "Order Materials" on the right; scroll down to "Shopping Guide")

- www.cornucopia.org—ratings for eggs, dairy, and other food-brand information

ORGANIZATIONS YOU MIGHT CONSIDER SUPPORTING

- Farm to Consumer Legal Defense Fund http://www.farmtoconsumer.org/—Support the small farmers treating animals, the Earth, and people right!

- The Weston A. Price Foundation http://www.westonaprice.org—become part of the traditional-foods movement

- The Price-Pottenger Nutrition Foundation http://www.ppnf.org—support those who are preserving important research and information on traditional foods and health

- The Institute for Responsible Technology http://www.responsibletechnology.org/—help raise awareness regarding the outrageous GMO liberties being taken

- The National Vaccine Information Center http://www.nvic.org—support those who are fighting for vaccine rights

- Jamie Oliver's Food Revolution http://www.jamieoliver.com/us/foundation/jamies-food-revolution/sign-petition

Acknowledgments

With deep appreciation, I'd like to acknowledge the work of Sally Fallon Morell, who has rightly brought national attention to the research of Dr. Weston A. Price and others who have documented the healing and protective power of traditional foods. Too many to list here, but so many other researchers, authors, farmers, and real-foods advocates are deeply appreciated, as well. Additionally, my children are owed a debt of gratitude for their tolerance of "mom's always working on the book!" Julie and Loretta, my lactating friends, thanks again for your up-to-date insights. To *all* my parents—I'm grateful for your love, support, and help with the kids during this labor-intensive project. Dave, thanks for everything. Acknowledgments would not be complete without thanking my agent, Marilyn (so instrumental in making this dream come true); the entire Fair Winds team, particularly Jill; and of course—the ever-insightful editor: JK. And finally, Jenny, Kevin, Nathan, Andrea, Richard, Annette, Michelle H., Danny, and Michelle L.—our farmers—I can never thank you enough for helping me to nourish my children.

—K.G.

To my dad, thank you for your unwavering persistence, imagining and creating this path for me. Thanks also to my mom, for your overwhelming support, your clear thinking, and your voice. I wish I had listened to you sooner. To my husband, thanks for converting me back into a meat eater so many years ago and for having confidence in me, even when it didn't always make sense (nor cents) to you. To my children, thank you for being my teachers and my students. FYI: I give you permission to give up the teaching part and let my patients take over this role. To my patients and their parents, thank you for cherishing your children and for trusting in me. Continue to always trust your gut and listen to that internal voice of reason. It will keep you on the right path.

—K.E.

About the Authors

KELLY GENZLINGER has dedicated many years to the study of nutrition and foods' effects within the human body. She is a traditional-foods advocate in her community and is dedicated to promoting wellness for her family and nutritional clients. An author, speaker, and certified nutritional consultant, Kelly is proud to have changed the lives of countless children and adults with her teachings, guidance, and counsel related to whole, real, traditional foods. With a business background and three professional certifications in holistic health and nutrition, she is an avid researcher. Kelly's first book, *Sugar . . . Stop the Addiction*, addressed the national crisis of excessive sugar consumption. She has been a featured speaker at wellness symposiums and a guest on cable shows such as *Diabetes Countdown* and *The Bottom Line*. She lives in southeastern Michigan with her husband and three well-nourished and loving children.

DR. KATHERINE ERLICH, M.D., is a board-certified pediatrician who spent her first eleven years after residency in a large, conventional pediatric practice. Combining her extensive clinical experience with her curiosity as to what makes children sick and how to help them heal, Dr. Erlich opened Healing the Whole Child, PLLC, and now practices out of the largest holistic medical center in the Midwest. Dr. Erlich guides her patients to better health through an individualized medical approach, integrating nutrition, holistic philosophies, and traditional medicine. Dr. Erlich has been instrumental in supporting her school district's Wellness Committee, featured on the news, and has authored articles printed in several publications. She lives in Franklin, Michigan, with her husband and two children.

Index